Copernicus Books

Sparking Curiosity and Explaining the World

Drawing inspiration from their Renaissance namesake, Copernicus books revolve around scientific curiosity and discovery. Authored by experts from around the world, our books strive to break down barriers and make scientific knowledge more accessible to the public, tackling modern concepts and technologies in a nontechnical and engaging way. Copernicus books are always written with the lay reader in mind, offering introductory forays into different fields to show how the world of science is transforming our daily lives. From astronomy to medicine, business to biology, you will find herein an enriching collection of literature that answers your questions and inspires you to ask even more.

Sam Goldstein • Robert B. Brooks
Donna DiMaio Rooney • Molly Anthony

Finding the Calm Child Within

Raising Resilient Children with Disruptive Mood Dysregulation Disorder

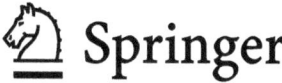

Sam Goldstein
School of Medicine
University of Utah
Salt Lake City, UT, USA

Donna DiMaio Rooney
Bethel, CT, USA

Robert B. Brooks
McLean Hospital
Needham, MA, USA

Molly Anthony
Plano, TX, USA

ISSN 2731-8982 ISSN 2731-8990 (electronic)
Copernicus Books
ISBN 978-3-031-90645-9 ISBN 978-3-031-90646-6 (eBook)
https://doi.org/10.1007/978-3-031-90646-6

© The Editor(s) (if applicable) and The Author(s), under exclusive license to Springer Nature Switzerland AG 2025

This work is subject to copyright. All rights are solely and exclusively licensed by the Publisher, whether the whole or part of the material is concerned, specifically the rights of translation, reprinting, reuse of illustrations, recitation, broadcasting, reproduction on microfilms or in any other physical way, and transmission or information storage and retrieval, electronic adaptation, computer software, or by similar or dissimilar methodology now known or hereafter developed.
The use of general descriptive names, registered names, trademarks, service marks, etc. in this publication does not imply, even in the absence of a specific statement, that such names are exempt from the relevant protective laws and regulations and therefore free for general use.
The publisher, the authors and the editors are safe to assume that the advice and information in this book are believed to be true and accurate at the date of publication. Neither the publisher nor the authors or the editors give a warranty, expressed or implied, with respect to the material contained herein or for any errors or omissions that may have been made. The publisher remains neutral with regard to jurisdictional claims in published maps and institutional affiliations.

This Springer imprint is published by the registered company Springer Nature Switzerland AG
The registered company address is: Gewerbestrasse 11, 6330 Cham, Switzerland

If disposing of this product, please recycle the paper.

Courage doesn't always roar. Sometimes, courage is the quiet voice at the end of the day saying, "I will try again tomorrow."
　　　　　　　　　　　　Mary Anne Radmacher

It does not matter how slowly you go, so long as you do not stop.
　　　　　　　　　　　　　　　　　Confucius

Perseverance is not a long race; it is many short races one after the other.
　　　　　　　　　　　　　　　Walter Elliot

The last thing to grow on a fruit tree is fruit.
　　　　　　　　　　　　　　　Tom Bilyeu

To the courageous families grappling with the daily challenges of raising a child with DMDD: may this serve as a beacon of hope, guidance, and strength, reminding you that resilience is not just possible but attainable. To the children whose emotional tempests inspire us to discover calm within ourselves, and to the parents whose love and dedication illuminate the path forward, you are seen, valued, and never alone on this journey.

Sam Goldstein

To the countless children and adolescents and their families who permitted me to enter their lives as a therapist, thank you. Working with you has reinforced my belief in the strength of human connections, empathy, persistence, and resilience when facing seemingly Herculean challenges. Thank you to my immediate family, Marilyn, Rich, Doug, Gigi, Suzanne, Maya, Teddy, Sophie, and Lyla, for enriching my life.

Robert Brooks

I dedicate this book to every parent and caregiver raising a child with DMDD. You are stronger than you think, as this disorder will test you in every possible way while enhancing your capacity to persevere. Hold on to hope, knowing that moments of calm can evolve into days of stability. A special thanks to my mom, Evelyn, for her relentless prayers and research, which guided us to Dr. Matthews. To Dr. Sol Lee, for graciously learning and prescribing the Matthews Protocol at my request. And to my husband, Jim, for I could not navigate this journey without you by my side.

Donna DiMaio Rooney

To my wonderful mother, Dee Dee, who has supported the search for stability for my son from day one. We couldn't have navigated life without you. To my fiancé, Bill, for his flexibility and unwavering support. Special thanks to Dr. Daniel Matthews and to the late Dr. Larry Fisher for dedicating their lives to helping children with DMDD break free from the chains that bind them and come to know true peace.

Molly Anthony

Acknowledgements

This book is dedicated to Dr. Joseph Biederman and Dr. Daniel Matthews, whose pioneering contributions to the study of mood disorders in children have brought hope and relief to families worldwide. Their relentless pursuit of knowledge and understanding has shaped how clinicians and researchers approach conditions like DMDD, providing critical insights and innovative solutions.

Dr. Biederman's groundbreaking research has redefined the landscape of child psychiatry, offering a clearer understanding of mood dysregulation and ensuring that children receive the urgent care they need. Dr. Matthews' compassionate clinical approach has been instrumental in guiding families through the complex emotional turmoil these disorders create, providing clarity and comfort.

Together, their work has revolutionized the field, delivering scientific breakthroughs and hope for children and families navigating these challenging conditions. Their legacy will continue to inspire future clinicians, researchers, and families.

Foreword

Fear, trepidation, isolation, and the immeasurable weight of guilt frequently plague most parents whose children suffer from Disruptive Mood Dysregulation Disorder (DMDD). The hallmark features of DMDD include frequent temper outbursts, chronic irritability, and angry moods, resulting in toxic interpersonal relationships and limited social problem-solving skills. Family life is often severely disrupted as anger and strife—coupled with aggression and rage—permeate most daily interactions. Oftentimes, parents are bewildered and perplexed as innocuous, benign situations pivot quickly toward bedlam and chaos. They may think, "What did I say to cause Billy to scream uncontrollably when I told him that he needs to make his bed in the morning? What did I say that made Jenny curse and throw a temper tantrum just because dinner was ready and it was time to wash up? What did I say to Chad that caused him to throw his phone and shatter its screen simply because I questioned the meaning of an inappropriate text he had sent to a friend?"

These severe emotional outbursts all have two things in common: first, the emotional intensity of the behavior and subsequent mood dysregulation are disproportionate to the context, and second, each parent assumed personal responsibility for the temper outbursts due to a misguided perception that behavior is the manifestation of a cause-and-effect paradigm. In other words, each parent inadvertently assumed that the trigger for their child's negative outburst was their own words and actions.

Perhaps no other endeavor is as challenging as parenting children in a consistent manner that fosters interpersonal growth and psychological maturity. Most of us—present author included—find ourselves ill-prepared and underqualified for the job demands inherent in this formidable task.

It is under this cloak of uncertainty and shadow of doubt that Robert Brooks and Sam Goldstein usher in a beacon of light wrapped in a four-letter word: hope. They don't offer any quick fixes, ubiquitous interventions, or majestic solutions to address the needs of children with deficits in mood dysregulation. Instead, these authors present core strategies and trove of suggestions to embolden families, allowing them to pursue thoughtful discussions aimed at preserving the dignity of both parents and children.

A consistent theme that resonates throughout each chapter is one of compassion (coupled with patience and understanding) for children who severely disrupt family life through their chronic outbursts and dysregulated behavior. This empathic approach also extends to parents, as co-authors Donna DiMaio Rooney and Molly Anthony provide engaging scenarios told from parents' perspectives that illustrate the intensity of the disorder, the perils of applying erroneous interventions to the disorder, and the fulfillment of even the smallest of wins.

The primary goal of Chap. 1 is to amplify the message that you are *not* alone—you'll read through three separate yet intertwined vignettes that demonstrate the challenges of raising a child with DMDD, the need for an accurate diagnosis, and the importance of a holistic intervention approach. Parenting is a journey! Knowing that a slew of mental health professionals are available to provide targeted services and family support groups provides the initial impetus that there is indeed hope.

Chapter 2 delves into the complexity of the disorder and what separates DMDD from other related emotional conditions (as well as how DMDD differs from ADHD). Due to a dearth of assessment instruments and the presence of frequent symptoms that overlap with other childhood conditions, diagnosing DMDD is tricky. The fact that DMDD is a relatively new condition further complicates the clinical picture—peer-reviewed literature on the prognoses and long-term outcomes (let alone the best practices in treatment regimens) remains somewhat limited.

The authors discuss the genesis of DMDD from various perspectives, including genetic predispositions, childhood temperament, neurotransmitter imbalances, and unsupportive environmental conditions during critical developmental periods. All of these factors intertwine in a manner that contributes to the chronic irritability, negative effects, and subsequent temper outbursts of children with DMDD. The chapter concludes with an important message echoed throughout the manuscript: *parents do not cause DMDD.*

Chapter 3 establishes the foundational principles and core standards for the remainder of the book by highlighting **eight essential guideposts** that serve as a kind of psychological GPS for parents. Each guidepost functions as an instructional edict, allowing parents to better understand their child's emotional volatility and to empower them by using negative setbacks as teachable moments that can foster emotional growth. Rather than offering a singular (and often impractical) solution to curb children's behavior dysregulation, the authors present a series of small but highly practical strategies whose cumulative weight can influence children toward gaining greater emotional stability. For example, modeling empathic behavior in everyday situations plays a crucial role in teaching children with DMDD how to better manage their emotions to solve social dilemmas.

Parents are encouraged to celebrate small successes as big victories, to encourage the use of "I" statements to take ownership of feelings, and to create a home environment that highlights a child's "islands of competence" in order to foster positive identity development. Throughout the chapter, the authors reiterate the power of unconditional love and acceptance, effective communication skills, and compassionate parenting during times of heightened family stress. Clearly, raising a child with DMDD requires more than typical parenting skills—parents must move beyond using pedestrian reinforcement systems to meet the unique and often unpredictable needs of their children who are afflicted with this disorder.

Chapter 8 might well be the most powerful chapter of the book—there, seeds of resilience are planted and cultivated as the authors explain how children can learn from rather than feel defined by their mistakes. In a world of helicopter mothers and bulldozer fathers who want to challenge school officials whenever their child makes a poor grade, challenge the coach whenever their child loses a ball game, or challenge their neighbor whenever another child may act untoward, it's refreshing to see the authors embrace a philosophy whereby childhood mistakes can serve as a catalyst for developing a growth mindset and ultimately resilience.

Resilience can be thought of as having the internal fortitude to emotionally and psychologically thrive in spite of the adversities, setbacks, and challenges that are inevitable in the journey of life. Everyone—children included—can establish resilience through cultivating a growth mindset, taking personal accountability for their actions, and using setbacks as teachable moments that can usher in a climate of change and learning from mistakes. This is much akin to the world of sports, wherein all good coaches stress to their players that resilient teams tend to learn more from a loss than a win.

We can all cultivate resilience by acknowledging and learning from our mistakes rather than blaming others or clinging to petty excuses. We can develop this resilience over time through adaptive coping strategies, supportive family systems, and a positive mindset. Simply put, resilience is the secret sauce in the pursuit of emotional wellness and psychological stability, especially for children with DMDD. It is the residue of the unconditional love that parents have for their children, and it is also the most precious gift that any parent can give their child—with resilience, children will be able to effectively manage future challenges because they'll be able to curb their frustrations and instead pursue rational decision-making.

Many books have been written about cultivating psychological wellness in children. Most, however, tend to follow a prescribed set of predetermined strategies or preach to parents from a rather haughty and conceited "top-down" perspective. The strength of *this* book lies in the writing style itself, as both Sam Goldstein and Robert Brooks model compassion and benevolence in the words they choose and tone in which these words are expressed. This is a book written for parents by expert clinicians in the fields of mental health and child development, who have unbridled respect for the demanding job of parenting, let alone parenting a child with DMDD.

The callout boxes provided by parents of children with DMDD, Molly Anthony and Donna DiMaio Rooney, provide a unique perspective on the trials and tribulations of the disorder. (Donna is also a founding member of Revolutionize DMDD.) There are no judgments, mandates, decrees, or authoritative edicts—instead, each chapter reiterates the need for supporting families to create a positive atmosphere where both children and parents can thrive. Poignant vignettes are woven into each chapter, which illustrate the techniques the authors recommend to subtly guide and steer parent–child interactions through turbulent waters.

DMDD is a complex disorder that can interrupt family dynamics and interpersonal relationships if not addressed in a holistic fashion. It takes a deft touch to write with this kind of care and sensitivity while simultaneously providing valuable insight and guidance for parents to raise emotionally resilient children. The pages that follow aren't just a trove of sound advice for parents of DMDD children, they're an astute collection of practical strategies will benefit *any* parent whose goals are to foster emotional wellness, enhance psychological resilience, and establish a growth mindset throughout their child's journey into adulthood.

Steven G. Feifer, D.Ed.
November 13th, 2024
Frederick, MD, USA
Author of *The Neuropsychology of Stress & Trauma: How to Develop a Trauma-Informed School*

Preface from Goldstein and Brooks

In the shadow of World War II, February 1944 was a time of intense military activity and national resolve in England. The nation was deeply engrossed in the war effort, with every facet of life impacted by the looming conflict. Amid the backdrop of this global turmoil, life in England continued with a sense of grim determination. Yet while the nation braced itself for the D-Day landings that would soon unfold on the shores of Normandy, another struggle was quietly being observed and recorded—one that would not reach its complete understanding until decades later.

Four months prior, Dr. Denis Hill, writing in the Proceedings of the Royal Society of Medicine, described a perplexing condition he termed "cerebral dysrhythmia." His observations centered on a group of children who exhibited violent, aggressive behaviors and prolonged, intense emotional outbursts. He proposed that these children were suffering from a neurological disorder, likely reflected in abnormal brain activity. Today, with the benefit of over 70 years of scientific advancement, we recognize that the condition Dr. Hill described bears striking similarities to what we now diagnose as Disruptive Mood Dysregulation Disorder (DMDD). His theory, though groundbreaking for its time, missed the mark in fully understanding the complex interplay of factors that contribute to this challenging disorder.

Parenting under any circumstances is a journey filled with unexpected challenges and profound joys. For those raising children with DMDD, though, this journey can often feel akin to navigating a relentless storm without a compass. We've crafted this book to be a guiding light for parents, caregivers, educators, and mental health professionals as they journey along the path toward understanding, supporting, and advocating for children affected by DMDD.

DMDD is a condition that challenges the very fabric of traditional parenting and educational techniques. Characterized by extreme irritability, anger, and frequent and intense temper outbursts, DMDD significantly impairs a child's ability to function in everyday life. Understanding the origins of DMDD is the first step toward demystifying this disorder. Through the real-life narratives of families raising children with DMDD, readers of this book will gain insights into the emotional resilience required to navigate the unique challenges posed by this condition. These stories will also demonstrate the profound impact that developing an emotionally resilient mindset can have on a child's growth and overall well-being. Our coauthors and parents of children with DMDD, Molly Anthony and Donna DiMaio Rooney, also provide a wealth of insights, experiences, and practical ideas in callout boxes titled "Parent's Perspective" throughout the book.

Beneath the surface of DMDD's turbulent expressions lies a complex interplay of biological, psychological, and environmental factors. Our book delves into the biological underpinnings of DMDD, offering a comprehensive understanding of its roots and presenting strategies for raising emotionally resilient children in this context. Recognizing the symptoms of DMDD and understanding the assessment process is crucial for securing the support and resources necessary for effective management and intervention. A formal diagnosis often marks a critical turning point, opening doors to specialized psychiatric interventions, counseling, and therapeutic strategies tailored to meet the unique needs of these children. In these pages, we provide a thorough overview of these interventions, emphasizing the importance of empathy, active listening, and unconditional love in fostering a nurturing and resilient home environment.

Parent training and medications for children are the cornerstone of effective DMDD management—together, they equip families with the tools and strategies that will create a supportive and understanding home atmosphere. Similarly, effective school interventions and advocacy are vital elements for making certain that children with DMDD receive the educational support and accommodations they need to be successful. Strengthening alliances between parents and schools is likewise another critical component for the healthy development of children with DMDD. Such alliances ensure that these children will be equipped with the skills, values, and self-discipline they'll need for fulfilling and productive lives. We devote an entire chapter to building an effective home/school alliance.

Finding the Calm Child Within represents a unique collaboration that bridges lived experiences with professional expertise. Co-authored by two parents who are intimately familiar with the day-to-day realities of raising children diagnosed with DMDD, this book offers a multifaceted perspective on a complex condition. Molly Anthony and Donna DiMaio Rooney bring authentic, deeply personal insights into the emotional roller coaster that their families and others in the DMDD community have endured. The featured families share a key quality: their never-ending quest to find answers to help their children. Readers will identify with many of the true stories woven throughout the book and will be able to learn from those who have emerged from having been deep in the trenches. The partnership between the four authors embodies the core message of this book: through collaboration, understanding, and dedicated support, it is possible to find calm amid the storm of DMDD.

To shed further light on this complicated disorder, we provide readers with a comprehensive knowledge of DMDD, from its clinical manifestations to cutting-edge therapeutic interventions. Our book builds upon a foundation of previous works that have explored the essential elements of resilience and self-discipline in children, including *Raising Resilient Children* and *Raising a Self-Disciplined Child*, both authored by Sam and Robert. These books have contributed to a generation of parents and educators understanding how to foster resilience in children who are facing various challenges. Additionally, their co-edited *Handbook of Resilience in Children* (first, second, and third editions) represents an in-depth exploration of the resilient mindset, offering theoretical and practical guidance for professionals in the field.

In writing *Finding the Calm Child Within*, we have sought to integrate the concepts of resilience and self-discipline within the context of DMDD, offering parents and professionals a comprehensive guide to understanding and managing this complex condition. We have focused upon eight guidelines that can be used to build and develop emotional health and resilience in children with DMDD. But our book is more than a parent handbook on managing DMDD, it's a testament to the resilience of the human spirit! It's a narrative of hope, highlighting the potential for growth, understanding, and transformation even in the face of significant challenges. We dedicate this book to all the families, educators, and professionals who are committed to the well-being and development of children with DMDD. Together, we can guide these children toward a promising, understanding, and compassionate future.

In these pages, parents will find strategies, knowledge, a community of support, and a testament to the strength of shared experiences. Parents will also discover the power that love and understanding have to illuminate even the darkest storms. Welcome to a journey of discovery, resilience, and hope!

Salt Lake City, UT, USA	Sam Goldstein
Needham, MA, USA	Robert B. Brooks

Preface from Anthony and Rooney

Parenting a child with DMDD comes with unique challenges and profound heartache. Yet it also fosters a deep desire—parents don't just want their child to thrive, they want *every* child living with this complex mood disorder to flourish. This shared experience creates an unspoken bond within the DMDD community, where parents support one another through the highs and lows.

Online DMDD support groups have become sanctuaries of solidarity and encouragement. Within these virtual spaces, parents celebrate even the most minor of victories, victories that might seem insignificant to the outside world but carry enormous weight for families navigating DMDD. These groups embody a spirit of collaboration, with parents lifting each other out of the trenches by sharing hard-earned wisdom and lessons learned.

The enduring words of the British philosopher Francis Bacon, "Knowledge is power," echo profoundly in this context. For parents of children with DMDD, knowledge doesn't just equate to power, it often serves as a lifeline. Many parents dive deeply into research, drawing insights from medical literature, expert advice, and personal trial and error. They then share this wealth of knowledge selflessly with others, united by a common goal: to help their own children and in turn to help other families navigating similar struggles.

The collective wisdom of these parents offers invaluable guidance, not as professional medical advice but as lived experiences. Every story shared, every bit of advice given holds the potential to light the way for another family. These true-life discoveries have proven transformative for the families we've featured in this book and can also provide hope and actionable insights for others.

Throughout these pages, you'll find honest advice from parents. Their stories are bound together by a common thread: through perseverance and shared learning, they've found strategies that work for their child with DMDD. While these experiences are not a substitute for professional guidance, they may serve as stepping stones toward a better future for others who are on a similar journey.

Bethel, CT, USA	Donna DiMaio Rooney
Plano, TX, USA	Molly Anthony

Praise for Finding the Calm Child Within

The authors blend professional expertise with parents' experiences to tackle DMDD. This book offers hope, practical solutions, and strategies to harness resilience, empowering families to navigate DMDD and make meaningful improvements in their children's lives. It will make a meaningful difference in my patients' lives.

—Judith Gooch M.D.

This book provides a welcome handle on a set of behaviors, first difficult to grasp, that may leave some at a loss. Its authors' expert voices and collective experiences lend a helping and reassuring hand to caregivers of children diagnosed with DMDD.

—Paul Stein, Ed.D., Executive Director, Schools for Children

Parenting confident, resilient children is challenging, especially when emotional regulation is a struggle. This expert guide on DMDD and resilience offers clear insights, practical strategies, and tools to empower parents. It prepares families to overcome challenges and nurture children into thriving, robust individuals—an invaluable resource for every parent.

—Bengi Semerci M.D.

Finding the Calm Child Within deepened my understanding of DDMD and inspired personal growth. The real-life stories and clear explanations highlighted ways to foster empathy and inclusion. The book underscores the transformative power of supportive adults in shaping resilient, confident children. I am grateful to the authors for their invaluable insights.

—Encarni Gallardo, MBA, CPM, Executive Director, Children's Service Society of Utah

This book is a powerful resource with expert insights and heartfelt wisdom. It equips parents to understand their child's unique needs, refine their parenting approach, and confidently advocate. It's a must-have tool. I'll gladly recommend it to the families I coach.
—Jami Kirkbride, Calm Connection Parenting Podcaster and Coach

This book is a vital resource for understanding DMDD. The authors expertly connect research, family dynamics, and practical interventions, emphasizing empathetic, communicative environments. Essential for clinicians and educators, it equips readers to address genetic, neurobiological, and environmental influences while fostering thriving children. This book is a must-read.
—Katie A. Dockweiler, Ed.D., NCSP, Co-founder, Healthy Minds, Safe Schools

This book is a game-changer for families and professionals. Through relatable narratives and practical strategies, it demystifies DMDD and empowers readers to differentiate it from other disorders. A must-read for building resilience and hope, it blends expert insights with compassionate guidance for thriving children and families.
—Alison G. Clark, Ed.S., NCSP, Co-founder, Healthy Minds Safe Schools

As a mother of a child whose life has been changed forever by the Matthews Protocol, this book is exactly what I wish I had access to when desperately looking for help, support, and answers. The Matthews Protocol described in this book saved our family and gave my child a future. For struggling parents of DMDD children, this book can be a life-changing guide.
—Brandi Waters, Parent of a child with DMDD

This insightful, accessible book turns the latest research on neuroscience and DMDD into valuable and practical advice for parents. It's a must-read for anyone interested in developing the tools for parenting a child with this complex condition.
—Nick Tsandes, LCSW

This book offers valuable insights and treatment protocols for children with emotional outbursts and Disruptive Mood Dysregulation Disorder (DMDD). It combines cutting-edge research with practical solutions, emphasizing that help is available and reminding readers they are not alone in navigating their child's emotional and psychological challenges.
—Nate, Major Dad Podcast

This book offers a compassionate exploration of the collaboration required when raising resilient children with Disruptive Mood Dysregulation Disorder. The authors present a positive perspective on strategies that can be employed by parents, educators, and clinicians alike. This book will serve as a beacon of light on your bookshelf.
—Karen E. Steves, MS, MBA, Co-director, Pathways Academy, McLean Hospital

Finding the Calm Child Within is an extraordinary resource for families and professionals. The reflections of real families who have overcome what many said was impossible lend a guiding light to families struggling with DMDD. The impact this could have on the psychiatric community is immeasurable.

—Jacqueline Mines, parent

This book is a lifeline for families navigating the challenges of raising children with complex emotional and behavioral needs. With practical strategies, evidence-based insights, and heartfelt compassion, it empowers parents to foster resilience, build strong connections, and create nurturing environments where their children can truly thrive. The author's work is a beacon of hope for families like mine.

—Corrie Zimerla, parent and Associate Dean of Operations, CWRU School of Medicine

This comprehensive and refreshing guide to DMDD looks beyond the child to the family system. The pages are filled with relatable stories and practical application points that empower struggling families on how to both raise a resilient child with DMDD and thrive as caregivers. I was impressed with the emphasis on empathy and caregivers, especially since we did so much of that work, including active listening, these past two years as a family. I only wish we had learned those skills earlier.

—Sara Patterson, parent of a child with DMDD

As a parent and professional, *Finding the Calm Child Within* deeply resonated with me. Written in a jargon-free, hopeful style, this informative book connects with parents and professionals seeking to understand and support kids with DMDD. The "eight guideposts" the authors present offer foundational strategies for helping kids tap into their strengths and resilience. While tailored for those dealing with DMDD, these guideposts can benefit all parents raising secure, resilient children.

—Charlie Appelstein, MSW, Author of *No Such Thing as a Bad Kid* & *The Gus Chronicles*

Finding the Calm Child Within is an essential guide for clinicians and parents. Blending expert insights with real-world parental perspectives, it offers practical strategies for supporting children with DMDD, managing emotional challenges, and fostering resilience. This collaborative resource is relatable, actionable, and invaluable for understanding and addressing the needs of children with this complex disorder—a must-read for building effective support strategies.

—Steven Baron, Psy.D., Psychologist, Author of *Teaching With A Strength-Based Approach: How To Motivate Students And Build Relationships*.

Finding the Calm Child Within expertly combines cutting-edge research, practical strategies, and real-life stories to illuminate DMDD. With clear insights for parents and clinicians, it offers invaluable guidance on building resilience and understanding this complex condition. Accessible and empowering, it's an essential read for anyone navigating or supporting someone through the challenges of DMDD.

—Caren Baruch-Feldman, Ph.D., Psychologist and Author of *The Grit Guide for Teens* and Co-Author of *The Resilience Workbook for Kids*

Finding the Calm Child Within is thoughtfully designed. Its combination of research data, the opinions of two experts in the field, and the expertise of mothers raising children with DMDD gives it depth and texture not commonly found in books written for a lay audience. The authors provide hopeful messages, helpful strategies, and a clear path for parents to feel encouraged and effective when raising their children. Educators, therapists, and parents alike will benefit from this incredible resource.

—Fairlee C. Fabrett, PhD, Director of Psychology Training, Child/Adolescent Division, McLean Hospital

With equal parts wisdom and warmth, *Finding the Calm Child Within* offers exceptional insight into best practices for supporting the development of resiliency in children and adolescents who struggle with dysregulation. It is clearly a must-read for clinicians and parents, and special education teachers and school administrators will also find it invaluable.

—Laura Mead, MS. Ed., Co-director, Pathways Academy, McLean Hospital

This is a groundbreaking resource for parents and caregivers of children diagnosed with DMDD. I wish I had had this information to consult when my twins were diagnosed a decade ago. We do better when we know better; this guide can help parents achieve both!

—Kathleen Barlow, founder of "Swimming UpScreen"

Contents

1	**The First Steps in Understanding DMDD**	1
	When Ordinary Parenting Strategies Fail	2
	Recognizing When Something Is Wrong	3
	The Emotional Toll on Families	4
	The First Steps to Seeking Help	5
	Raising Resilient Children with DMDD	7
	Final Words	9
2	**Understanding DMDD**	11
	Ben's Story	11
	Overview and Symptoms of DMDD	12
	Diagnostic Criteria for DMDD	13
	Recurrent and Severe Temper Tantrums or Outbursts	13
	Persistent Irritability or Anger	13
	Duration of Symptoms	14
	Onset of Symptoms	14
	Settings	14
	Age of Onset	15
	Exclusion of Other Disorders	15
	The Developmental Roots of DMDD	15
	Early Childhood Development	16
	Contributing Factors to DMDD	17
	Genetic Factors	17
	Neurobiological Factors	17
	Environmental Factors	18
	Cumulative Impact	19
	Timing and Developmental Milestones	19
	Co-occurring Problems in DMDD	20
	ADHD and DMDD	20
	Anxiety Disorders and DMDD	22
	Oppositional Defiant Disorder (ODD) and DMDD	22

Major Depression and DMDD 23
Bipolar Disorder and DMDD 23
Intermittent Explosive Disorder and DMDD 24
Autism Spectrum Disorder (ASD) and DMDD 24
Implications for Treatment of Co-occurring Conditions 25
Ben's Story Continues... 26
Implications for Treatment and Intervention 27
Pharmacotherapy... 27
The Matthews Protocol..................................... 28
Cognitive-Behavioral Therapy (CBT) 31
Parent Training and Family Therapy.......................... 32
School-Based Interventions 32
Early Intervention 32
A Holistic Approach 33
The Bottom Line.. 33
Final Words... 34

3 The Eight Guideposts for Raising Emotionally Resilient Children with DMDD 35
Jonas' Story... 35
Teaching and Conveying Empathy 36
Effective Communication and Listening Actively 37
Accepting Children for Who They Are: Conveying Unconditional Love and Setting Realistic Expectations......................... 38
Nurturing "Islands of Competence" 40
Helping Children Learn from Rather Than Feel Defeated by Mistakes... 41
Teaching Children to Solve Problems and Make Sound Decisions 42
Disciplining in Ways That Promote Self-Discipline and Self-Worth ... 43
Developing Responsibility, Compassion, and a Social Conscience 45
Returning to Jonas.. 47
Final Thoughts and a Cautionary Note........................... 47

4 Teaching and Conveying Empathy to Children with DMDD 51
Patrick's Story.. 51
The Importance of Empathy in Raising Resilient Children 53
Modeling Empathy: A Parent's Role 53
Active Listening 54
Reflecting Feelings 54
Demonstrating Patience 55
Teaching Empathy to Children with DMDD 56
Labeling Emotions 56
Role-Playing... 57
Encouraging Perspective-Taking 58
Praising Empathic Behavior................................ 58
Storytelling and Books 59
The Struggle for Parents to Remain Empathic 60

	Feeling Stressed and Overwhelmed	60
	Fatigue	61
	Defensive Reactions	61
	Inconsistent Boundaries	62
	Past Parenting Experiences and Guilt	62
	Significant Disciplinary Differences Between Parents	63
	Additional Strategies to Overcome Obstacles to Empathy	64
	Self-Care	64
	Seeking Support	64
	Mindfulness Practices	65
	A Few Words About Siblings	66
	Back to Patrick	67
	Final Words	68
5	**Effective Communication and Listening Actively**	69
	Bella and Lizzie's Story	69
	Reflecting on Communication: A Path to Fostering Resilience in Children	70
	Questions to Evaluate Communication Practices	70
	The Role of Communication in Managing DMDD	75
	Strategies for Improving Communication	76
	Active Listening: Fully Engaging with Your Child	76
	Validation: Acknowledging Your Child's Emotions	77
	Setting Boundaries with Compassion: Balancing Limits and Empathy	77
	Modeling Emotional Regulation: Teaching by Example	78
	Finding Solutions to Challenges and Obstacles	79
	Returning to the Twins	82
	Conclusion: Building Stronger Family Connections	83
6	**Accepting Our Children for Who They Are: Conveying Unconditional Love and Setting Realistic Expectations**	85
	Barry's Story	85
	The Importance of Unconditional Love	86
	Demonstrating Unconditional Love	87
	Consistent Emotional Support	88
	Expressing Affection Through Nonverbal Cues	88
	Reassurance and Validation of Emotions	89
	Creating Safe, Predictable Routines	89
	Spending Quality One-on-One Time Together	90
	Setting Realistic Expectations	90
	Adjusting Expectations with Compassion	91
	Breaking Down Larger Goals into Smaller Steps	91
	Modeling Flexibility in Expectations	92
	Encouraging Effort Over Outcome	92
	Celebrating Strengths	92

	Identifying and Reinforcing Strengths	93
	Offering Opportunities to Shine in Their Strengths	93
	Compassionately Addressing Difficulties	94
	Exploring the Root Cause of Behavior	94
	Using Reflective Listening	95
	Fostering a Supportive Environment	95
	Creating an Emotional Safe Haven	96
	Encouraging Open Communication	97
	Challenges to Acceptance and How to Overcome Them	97
	Emotional Exhaustion and Burnout	97
	Difficulty with Communication	98
	Public Meltdowns and Social Stigma	99
	Let's Return to Barry	101
	Maintaining Consistency in Routines	102
	Key Takeaways	102
7	**Nurturing "Islands of Competence"**	105
	Zack and Annie's Story	105
	Understanding the Origins of "Islands of Competence"	107
	Strategies for Nurturing "Islands of Competence"	108
	Recognize and Celebrate Small Successes	109
	Create Opportunities for Mastery	110
	Set Realistic Expectations and Celebrate Effort	111
	Encourage Social Reinforcement	113
	Model Emotional Resilience Through "Islands of Competence"	115
	Challenges in "Nurturing Islands of Competence"	116
	Navigating Behavioral Challenges	116
	Balancing Competence with Academic Expectations: The Role of Islands of Competence	119
	Focusing Too Much on Competence: The Balance Between Nurturing Strengths and Encouraging Growth	120
	Returning to Zack and Annie's Story	122
	Key Takeaways	123
8	**Helping Children with DMDD Learn from, Rather Than Feel Defeated by Mistakes**	125
	Kellan's Story	125
	The Growth Mindset: A Path to Resilience	127
	Understanding the Impact of DMDD on Mindset	128
	The Role of a Growth Mindset in Emotional Regulation	128
	Encouraging a Growth Mindset in Children with DMDD	129
	Modeling a Growth Mindset in Everyday Interactions	129
	Praising Effort Over Outcomes	130
	Encouraging Realistic Risk-Taking and Learning from Mistakes	131
	Reframing Mistakes as Learning Opportunities	132

	Teaching Self-Compassion	132
	Engaging in Reflective Questioning	133
	Normalizing Mistakes in the Family Culture	134
	Creating Opportunities for Controlled Risk-Taking	134
	Why Mistakes Can Feel So Catastrophic	135
	Obstacles to Helping Children Learn from Mistakes	135
	Temperament and Emotional Sensitivity	136
	Adverse Parental Reactions to Mistakes	137
	Social Comparisons and External Pressure	138
	Lack of Immediate Solutions	139
	Back to Kellan's Story	139
	The Long-Term Impact of a Growth Mindset	140
9	**The Importance of Problem-Solving and Decision-Making Skills for Children with DMDD**	**143**
	Joseph's Story	143
	The Unique Challenges of Problem-Solving for Children with DMDD	145
	Step 1: Identify the Problem	145
	Step 2: Brainstorm Solutions	146
	Step 3: Weigh the Pros and Cons	147
	Step 4: Implement the Decision	147
	Step 5: Monitor and Reflect on the Outcome	148
	Step 6: Reinforce Independence and Confidence	149
	Practical Exercises for Problem-Solving and Decision-Making	149
	Exercise 1: The Decision-Making Jar	149
	Exercise 2: The Problem-Solving Chart	150
	Exercise 3: The "What If?" Game	150
	Exercise 4: The Emotion Thermometer	151
	Common Obstacles to Problem-Solving and Decision-Making	151
	Obstacle 1: Emotional Overload	151
	Obstacle 2: Perfectionism	152
	Obstacle 3: Impulsivity	152
	Obstacle 4: Lack of Confidence	153
	Building Resilience Through Problem-Solving	153
	Real-Life Applications for Parents	154
	Encouraging Decision-Making in Everyday Situations	154
	Normalizing Mistakes to Alleviate Anxiety	155
	Practicing Problem-Solving During Family Discussions	155
	Using Visual Aids and Tools	156
	Praising Effort Over Outcomes	157
	The Long-Term Benefits of Teaching Problem-Solving and Decision-Making	157
	Final Words	157

10 Disciplining in Ways that Promote Self-Discipline and Self-Worth ... 159
Nathan's Story. ... 159
The Role of Discipline in Building Resilience ... 163
Shifting the Focus: From Punishment to Emotional Growth ... 163
Developing Emotional Intelligence and Problem-Solving Skills ... 164
Building a Resilient Mindset ... 164
Discipline as a Foundation for Resilience ... 165
Understanding DMDD and the Role of Discipline. ... 165
Positive Reinforcement: Building on Strengths ... 166
Implementing Positive Reinforcement ... 166
Consistency in Rules and Expectations ... 167
Six Strategies for Promoting Self-Discipline ... 168
    Emotional Regulation Before Consequence-Based Discipline. ... 168
    Consistent Routines to Reduce Anxiety ... 169
Response Cost: Empowering Children with DMDD to Maintain Positive Behaviors. ... 169
Empathy and Emotional Validation ... 170
A Problem-Solving Approach. ... 171
Teaching Coping Skills. ... 171
Obstacles and Solutions in Discipline. ... 172
    Punitive Discipline ... 172
    The Dangers of Negative Reinforcement ... 172
    Parent Burnout ... 173
    Slow Is Not Fast Enough ... 173
    Hypersensitivity ... 174
Addressing the Underlying Reasons for Challenging Behavior. ... 175
Empathy: The Key to Effective Discipline ... 175
Conclusion: Discipline as a Tool for Growth ... 176

11 Developing Responsibility, Compassion, and a Social Conscience... 177
Ethan's Story. ... 177
Nurturing Responsibility Through Positive Engagement. ... 179
Creating a Rewarding Framework for Contribution. ... 180
Encouraging Consistent Reflection on Contributions. ... 182
The Power of Compassion in Developing a Social Conscience. ... 183
Broadening Compassion Through Exposure to Diverse Experiences ... 184
Modeling Compassionate Behavior ... 184
Overcoming Obstacles in Teaching Responsibility and Compassion. ... 185
    Implementing Collaborative Problem-Solving. ... 186
    Teaching Self-Regulation and Emotional Management. ... 187
Conclusion: The Path to Responsibility, Compassion, and Social Conscience ... 188

Contents · xxxi

12 Establishing a Partnership with Your Child's School 189
Emma's Story 189
    Emotional Regulation Strategies 190
    Structured Routines 190
    Positive Reinforcement 191
    Frequent Check-Ins 191
    Parent Involvement 191
How the Brain Learns 193
    Ability 193
    Knowledge 194
    Skill 194
The Unique Challenges of DMDD in School 194
The Role of Parents in the Educational Process 195
Expanding Parent Involvement: The Broader Impact 196
Addressing Barriers to Parental Involvement 197
The School's Role in Supporting Parental Involvement 198
Building Open Lines of Communication 198
Understanding School Policies and Procedures 199
Supporting a Child's Learning at Home 200
Overcoming Common Challenges in Parent-School Partnerships 200
    Differences in Communication Styles 200
    Solution 201
    Conflicting Schedules 201
    Solution 202
    Misunderstanding a Child's Behavior 202
    Solution 204
    Resolving Conflicts 204
    Solution 205
Celebrating Successes Together 206
Building a Collaborative Community 206
The Lasting Impacts of a Strong Parent-School Partnership 207

13 Rising Through the Storm 209
Similarities in Challenges: A Turbulent Journey 209
    Early Signs of Emotional Dysregulation 210
    Struggles with Misdiagnoses and Inadequate Treatments 211
    Behavioral Outbursts and the Impacts on Family Life 211
    Isolation and Misunderstanding 212
Rising Above the Challenges: Paths to Progress and Happiness 213
    Finding the Right Diagnosis 213
    Effective Treatment and Medication 214
    Supportive Relationships 215
    Personal Growth and Transformation 216
    Learning When to Act 216
Resilient Children with DMDD 217

    Embracing a Growth Mindset............................. 218
    Focusing on What *Can* Be Controlled 218
    The Role of Supportive Adults 219
    The Power of Hope...................................... 220
  The Dreams and Wishes of Parents........................... 220
  Words for the Professionals Who Work with Children with DMDD
  and Their Families 221
  Rising Through the Storm................................... 222

Appendix A 225

Appendix B 229

Resources... 235

Index... 239

Quick Solution Finder

Accepting Children for Who They Are, 7–8, 38–39

- Demonstrating Unconditional Love, 7, 87–90
- Setting Realistic and Attainable Expectations, 7, 38–39, 48, 71, 85–103, 111–113
- Celebrating Small Victories to Build Confidence, 48

Active Listening Techniques, 52, 54, 66, 76, 84

- Eliminating Distractions to Engage Fully, 54
- Using Open-Ended Questions to Foster Dialogue, 54
- Paraphrasing and Reflecting Feelings for Validation, 54–55
- Mindfulness Practices, 65–66

    - Incorporating meditation and breathing exercises to help children center themselves, 65
    - Practicing mindful communication to remain present during family interactions.

- The Importance of Unconditional Love, 86–87

    - Why love and acceptance are vital for children with DMDD, 86
    - Strategies for Demonstrating Unconditional Love, 87–90

        - Providing consistent emotional support, 88
        - Using nonverbal cues like touch and gestures, 88–89
        - Validating emotions and offering reassurance, 89
        - Creating predictable routines to reduce anxiety, 89–90
        - Spending quality one-on-one time to strengthen bonds, 90

ADHD (Co-occurring Disorder), 12, 13, 20–21, 25, 82, 85, 101, 106, 118, 122, 125, 143, 159, 160, 168, 177, 211, 213

Addressing Defensive Reactions, 61–62

- Depersonalizing a Child's Outbursts, 62
- Reframing Behavior as Symptoms, Not Personal Attacks, 62

Addressing Emotional Challenges, 94

- Dealing with Emotional Outbursts, 52
  - Providing space for the child to calm down independently, 79
  - Using follow-up conversations to address underlying causes, 81
  - Avoiding immediate problem-solving during heightened emotional states, 81

Addressing the Stigma Around DMDD Diagnosis and Treatment, 20
Alternative Medications and Their Uses, 30
Anxiety Disorders (Co-occurring Disorder), 22
Autism Spectrum Disorder (ASD), 7, 15, 24–25, 100, 159, 201, 204, 213
Balancing Behavioral Challenges with Positive Reinforcement, 172

- Addressing disruptive behaviors calmly and constructively.
- Highlighting and praising the child's positive actions and skills alongside setting clear behavioral boundaries.

Balancing Hope and Realistic Expectations in DMDD Treatment
Balancing Immediate Safety with Long-Term Empathic Responses

- Ensuring Safety During Emotional Outbursts
- Avoiding Escalation by Prioritizing Peaceful Periods, 49
- Using Setbacks as Opportunities for Growth and Understanding, 79

Behavioral and Psychotherapeutic Interventions, 24, 25, 177, 199, 220

- Cognitive-behavioral therapy (CBT), 9, 25, 31
- Parent Training Programs, 9, 16, 32
- Family Therapy Approaches, 10, 32, 65, 190

Building a Structured and Predictable Home Environment, 34
Building Confidence Through Adaptive Strategies, 132
Building Emotional Awareness in Parents and Children, 46
Building Resilience in Children, 8, 148, 164

- Encouraging a Growth Mindset, 129–135, 152
  - Emphasizing learning from mistakes as part of growth, 129–130
  - Praising effort rather than perfection, 130–131

Celebrating Empathy Publicly Within the Family, 59
Celebrating Small Victories in Emotional Regulation, 56
Collaborative Problem-Solving with Children, 58, 186–187
Compassionate Boundary-Setting, 77–78, 84

- Balancing empathy with clear expectations, 77
- Offering limited choices to empower the child, 72
- Using calm and respectful language when enforcing boundaries, 38
- Ensuring consistency in expectations without rigidity, 81

Quick Solution Finder

Connecting with Support Networks
Contributing Genetic Factors to DMDD, 17
Co-occurring Disorders and Their Impact, 25

- ADHD, 12, 13, 20–21, 25, 82, 85, 101, 106, 118, 122, 125, 143, 159, 160, 168, 177, 211, 213
- Anxiety Disorders, 22
- Oppositional Defiant Disorder (ODD), 13, 22–23, 25, 213
- Major Depression, 23
- Bipolar Disorder (BD), 12, 15, 23–24, 105, 125
- Intermittent Explosive Disorder (IED), 22, 24
- Autism Spectrum Disorder (ASD), 7, 15, 24–25, 100, 159, 201, 204, 213

Creating Opportunities for Mastery, 110
Creating Opportunities for Practicing Kindness, 7, 36
Demonstrating Patience, 55–56

- Using Mindful Breathing During Emotional Escalations, 55
- Celebrating Small Victories in Emotional Regulation, 55
- Balancing Immediate Safety with Long-Term Empathic Responses, 55

Developmental Roots of DMDD: Temperament and Early Attachment, 15
Diagnostic Criteria for DMDD, 12–15, 22, 24, 25, 33, 177
Dietary and Lifestyle Influences on DMDD Symptoms, 18, 19
Disciplining to Promote Self-Discipline and Self-Worth, 8, 43–45, 48, 159–176

- Using Positive Reinforcement Instead of Punishment, 166
- Implementing Natural and Logical Consequences, 44
- Maintaining Dignity During Disciplinary Moments, 44

DMDD vs. PANS/PANDAS: Recognizing Rapid-Onset Symptoms, 14
Early Recognition and Diagnosis of DMDD, 19
Effective Communication and Active Listening, 7, 37–38, 48, 69–84

- Techniques for Engaged Listening, 54
- Validating Emotions to Foster Trust, 7
- Teaching Constructive Expression of Feelings, 38
- Empathy as a Cornerstone of Emotional Resilience, 7, 36, 52
- Modeling Empathy in Daily Interactions, 7
- Creating Opportunities for Practicing Kindness, 7, 36
- Using Transparency to Normalize Emotional Experiences, 37, 41

Encouraging Exploration of New Interests, 107
Encouraging Perspective-Taking, 58

- Asking Reflective Questions About Others' Feelings, 133–134
- Modeling Empathy in Real-Life Scenarios, 57

Ensuring Safety During Emotional Outbursts
Fostering Empathy and Connection, 53, 66, 74

- Teaching Empathy and Compassion, 71
    - Modeling understanding and kindness, 59
    - Highlighting how emotions affect others in the family, 57
    - Building an emotionally supportive family culture, 134

Family Therapy for DMDD, 32, 65
Final Insights on Empathy's Transformative Power, 68

- Empathy as the First Step in Building Resilience
- Integrating Empathy With Other Parenting Guideposts
- Setting the Stage for Future Skills: Communication, Problem-Solving, and Discipline

Fostering Responsibility, Compassion, and a Social Conscience, 178

- Involving Children in Community Service, 7, 9
- Teaching Accountability for Actions, 46
- Cultivating Awareness of Broader Social Issues

Frequent and Intense Emotional Outbursts, 52, 137, 143, 172, 221
Guiding Rather Than Solving, 171

- Helping children identify problems and potential solutions, 8, 164
- Encouraging independent problem-solving to build confidence, 42, 71

Impact of DMDD on Family Dynamics, 32, 83
Importance of Early Intervention for DMDD, 20, 32
Implementing Structured Routines, 169, 190

- Using visual schedules to create predictability, 190
- Preparing children for transitions with advance notice, 190

Inconsistent Boundaries, 62
Intermittent Explosive Disorder (IED), 22, 24
Labeling Emotions, 56–57

- Using Emotion Charts and Visual Aids, 56
- Modeling Emotion Labeling in Everyday Life, 57

Learning About DMDD and Related Conditions, 12, 20, 24–26, 107, 168, 192, 198, 221
Leveraging Strengths to Build Confidence, 109

- Showcasing and celebrating achievements in areas where the child feels competent, 109
- Using visual reminders of successes, like displaying artwork or completed projects, to reinforce confidence, 109

Long-Term Outlook for Children with DMDD, 26, 32, 33, 94
Maintaining Compassion While Enforcing Rules, 226
Managing Emotional Strain in Sibling Relationships, 66
Managing Puberty and Hormonal Changes in DMDD, 30
Managing Stress and Feeling Overwhelmed, 60–61

- Techniques for Decompressing After Stressful Moments, 60
- Building a Toolbox of Quick Self-Calming Strategies, 60

Matthews Protocol and Its Implementation, 177
Medication Interventions and the Matthews Protocol, 26, 28–30

- Exploring Medication Options and Transitions, 28
- Combining Pharmacotherapy With Behavioral Strategies, 27
- Understanding the Role of Flexible Medication Approaches

Modeling Empathy: Parental Strategies, 53–56

- Active Listening Techniques, 52, 54, 66, 76, 84
- Reflecting Feelings, 52–55
- Demonstrating Patience, 55–56

Navigating Crisis Situations in DMDD, 39, 48

- Strategies for Immediate Intervention
- Balancing Calm and Decisive Actions During Crises, 217
- Preserving Peace in Fragile Situations, 49

Navigating Misdiagnoses and Medication Challenges, 211
Neurobiological Underpinnings of DMDD, 17–18, 27
Nurturing "Islands of Competence", 8, 40–41, 105–124

- Identifying and Cultivating Strengths, 8, 93, 206
- Creating Opportunities for Success, 110
- Encouraging Exploration of New Interests, 107

Oppositional Defiant Disorder (ODD), 13, 22–23, 25, 213
Ordinary Parenting Strategies Fail, 2–3
Overcoming Obstacles to Empathy for Parents, 60–63

- Managing Stress and Feeling Overwhelmed, 60–61
- Coping with Fatigue, 61
- Addressing Defensive Reactions, 61–62
- Navigating Inconsistent Boundaries, 62
- Dealing With Guilt or Past Parenting Challenges, 62–63
- Resolving Parental Disciplinary Differences, 63

Parenting Flexibility and Adaptability, 49
Parenting Support Programs for Mood Disorders, 32
Praising Empathic Behavior, 58–59

- Using Specific Praise to Reinforce Positive Actions, 58, 59

Problem-solving and Decision-Making Skills, 43, 143–158

- Structured Framework for Tackling Problems, 144
- Teaching Evaluation of Options and Consequences, 8, 43
- Encouraging Reflective Practices to Assess Outcomes, 182

Recognizing Patterns of Persistent Irritability, 13
Reducing the Emotional Toll on Families, 4
Reflecting Feelings, 52–55

- Observing Verbal and Nonverbal Cues, 55
- Building Emotional Vocabulary for Children, 55

Resolving Parental Disciplinary Differences, 63
Role-Playing Activities, 57

- Practicing Perspective-Taking Through Relatable Scenarios, 57
- Using Puppets or Toys to Act Out Emotional Situations, 57

School-Based Interventions for Children with DMDD, 32, 33
Seeking Professional Help, 5, 214
Self-Care Strategies for Parents, 34, 52, 60, 64, 98, 173
Setting Realistic and Attainable Expectations, 7, 38–39, 48, 71, 85–103, 111–113
Signs and Symptoms of DMDD, 9, 12–16, 18, 19, 21, 23–25, 28–30, 34, 204, 220
Stigma of Seeking Mental Health Help, 6
Stories of Transformation Through Empathy, 48, 214–216
Teaching Accountability for Actions, 46
Teaching Children to Learn From Mistakes, 135–139, 141

- Adopting a Growth Mindset, 128, 218
- Reflective Practices for Analyzing Actions, 182
- Fostering Resilience Through Encouragement and Support, 93, 130, 131, 191, 213, 219

Teaching Constructive Expression of Feelings, 38
Teaching Empathy to Children with DMDD, 36, 56–60
Teaching Evaluation of Options and Consequences, 8, 43
Temper Outbursts and Persistent Irritability, 15
The Role of Empathy in Supporting Emotional Resilience, 7, 36, 52, 53
Understanding Emotional Dysregulation, 6, 183
Understanding Mistakes as Learning Opportunities, 8, 41, 73, 132, 152

- Reframing mistakes as opportunities to grow, not failures, 127, 132
- Teaching children to see mistakes as temporary and solvable problems, 42

Understanding Onset and Duration of Symptoms, 14, 15
Using Setbacks as Opportunities for Growth and Understanding, 128, 148
Validating Emotions to Foster Trust, 7

About the Authors

Sam Goldstein, Ph.D. is a neuropsychologist specializing in school psychology, child development, and neuropsychology. Licensed in Utah, he is a certified Developmental Disabilities evaluator, board-certified Pediatric Neuropsychologist, and a Fellow of leading neuropsychology and cerebral palsy academies. He has served as Assistant Clinical Instructor in Psychiatry and has directed a private multidisciplinary team addressing neurological, learning, and behavioral issues since 1980. Dr. Goldstein is on staff at the University Neuropsychiatric Institute and has contributed to the Craniofacial Team and Developmental Disabilities Clinic at the University of Utah. A prolific author, Dr. Goldstein has written or edited over 50 publications, including 21 textbooks on behavior, ADHD, resilience, and learning disabilities, and the *Clinician Guide to Disruptive Mood Dysregulation Disorder* (2024). He has developed a dozen psychological tests. He has also collaborated extensively, producing seminal works on resilience, classroom management, autism, and neurodevelopmental disorders. Visit samgoldstein.com.

Robert Brooks, Ph.D. is a clinical psychologist and part-time faculty member at Harvard Medical School and former Director of Psychology at McLean Hospital. He is an expert on resilience, education, special needs, psychotherapy, parenting, and fostering positive environments. Dr. Brooks has authored or co-authored 22 books, 36 book chapters, and 36 peer-reviewed articles. He has received numerous awards, including Hall of Fame honors from the Connecticut Association of Children with LD and CHADD, the Mental Health Humanitarian Award from William James College, and the 2023 Trailblazer Award from Worldmaker International for his contributions to resilience. Dr. Brooks has consulted for Sesame Street Parents Magazine and continues to inspire through his lectures, writings, and groundbreaking work in mental health. Visit drrobertbrooks.com.

Donna DiMaio Rooney, a Pace University graduate (1990), began her career in television, contributing to shows like *LIVE! with Regis and Kathie Lee* and *Good Morning America*. Transitioning to public relations, she earned two silver HSMAI Golden Bell awards before venturing independently. She is an accomplished writer and has contributed to books and magazines, including *DANI and the Day the Bully Changed Everything*, which received a gold Mom's Choice Award®. Passionate about youth advocacy, she co-founded Revolutionize DMDD and co-authored a chapter in *Clinician Guide to Disruptive Mood Dysregulation Disorder in Children and Adolescents* (2024). Donna resides in Connecticut with her family and their Shih-Poo.

Molly Anthony, a Brigham Young University graduate with a Bachelor of Fine Arts, began her career as a graphic designer before transitioning to the medical field as a certified medical assistant at an ADHD clinic. A parent of a child with DMDD, she has dedicated her life to understanding the disorder and fostering stability. Growing up in a family with mood disorders and ADHD, Molly offers unique insights from both child and parent perspectives. In 2024, she co-authored *DMDD from the Front Line: The Parent's Perspective*, featured in the *Clinician Guide to Disruptive Mood Dysregulation Disorder in Children and Adolescents*.

Also by Goldstein and Brooks

Raising Resilient Children (2001)
Seven Steps to Help Your Child Worry Less (with Kristy Hagar) (2002)
Parenting Resilient Children Parent Training Manual (2002)
Nurturing Resilience in Our Children (2003)
The Power of Resilience (2004)
Angry Children, Worried Parents (with Sharon Weiss) (2004)
Handbook of Resilience in Children (2005)
Seven Steps to Improve Your Child's Social Skills (with Kristy Hagar) (2006)
Understanding and Managing Children's Classroom Behavior—2nd Edition (2007)
Raising a Self-Disciplined Child (2007)
Raising Resilient Children with Autism Spectrum Disorders (2012)
Handbook of Resilience in Children—2nd Edition (2012)
Play Therapy Interventions to Enhance Resilience (with David Crenshaw) (2015)
Tenacity in Children (2021)
Handbook of Resilience in Children—3rd Edition (2023)
Graham And Poppy's Quest for Tenacity (2024)

I Am DMDD

I am DMDD, a storm without end,
I twist in the mind where peace cannot mend.
Explosive outbursts, rage without cause,
Breaking the calm, a shark's iron jaws.

I live in the tantrums, in screams that won't cease,
Turning quiet moments into battles, no peace.
I flood every room with chaos and fear,
Drowning out laughter, the joy disappears.

I tear at the heartstrings of family and home,
Leaving everyone feeling lost and alone.
I hijack their smiles, replace them with tears,
Planting doubt in their minds, sowing endless fears.

But through all of the wreckage, all of the shame,
A glimmer of hope shines through the pain.
I am DMDD, but I can be defeated,
With love, strength, and knowledge, my hold is depleted.

Come closer, let me whisper in your ear.

—Sam Goldstein

Chapter 1
The First Steps in Understanding DMDD

It was a typical afternoon in the Brown household, with sunlight filtering through the curtains as eight-year-old Liam sat at the kitchen table, his face scrunched up in concentration over a math problem. What happened next would forever change the way his parents understood their child. Frustrated by a simple subtraction error, Liam's mood shifted abruptly, and within moments, a storm of emotions erupted. His screams filled the house, drowning out the peaceful hum of daily life—papers flew, a pencil snapped in half, and Liam's cries of frustration echoed through the rooms. His parents could only stand next to him helplessly, unsure of what to do or say.

This wasn't the first time Michael and Sarah had witnessed such an outburst—the frequency and severity of Liam's episodes had been escalating for months, leaving them feeling increasingly isolated and alarmed—but this episode was one of the most intense they'd seen. Michael and Sarah had always prided themselves on being the kind of parents who blended discipline and love, yet nothing they tried seemed to calm Liam during these outbursts. Quite the contrary: their usual strategies of time-outs, reasoning, and even comforting only heightened his distress.

> We have found DMDD to be very isolating. We've never met another child diagnosed with DMDD, nor have we met other parents who have dealt with this disorder. When strangers offer advice, it can often arrive at the worst times, such as when your child is in crisis. Frequently, I receive advice from middle-aged women who judge me as an inexperienced and incompetent dad who needs instruction. I'm not one of those dads, but my situation is too complicated to explain. It's a wonderful privilege to use the internet to connect with other parents worldwide who have children with chronic irritability. I've learned more from them than from any other source.

Across town, a similar scene was playing out in the Gupta household. Ten-year-old Anika, usually a bright and composed child, had spiraled into inconsolable distress after a minor disagreement with her older brother Arjun. What had started out as a typical sibling spat over a remote control quickly escalated into a full-blown meltdown. Anika's frustration was palpable; her parents felt a familiar knot of anxiety tighten in their stomachs as they watched her struggle to regain control. Raj and Priya had seen this pattern before, and each time it happened, it left them feeling more desperate for answers.

Meanwhile, the Morgan family was also grappling with an increasingly volatile situation in another part of the city. Seven-year-old Maya, once the sunshine of her family thanks to her infectious laughter and cheerful nature, had become prone to sudden fits of anger and irritability. That evening, as her mother Elena prepared dinner, a simple request to set the table triggered an outburst so fierce that Maya's small hands clenched into fists and her face turned red with rage. When her father David got home and walked into the kitchen, his heart sank. He had been trying to ignore the signs, hoping that Maya's behavior was just a phase, but deep down, he knew something more serious was happening.

Three different families, three different homes, yet the challenge was the same: how to understand and help a child whose emotions seemed to have taken on a life of their own? For the Browns, Guptas, and Morgans, these episodes weren't just about temper tantrums or misbehavior—they were signals of a deeper, more complex issue. But what could it be? How could they find the right way to help their children?

When Ordinary Parenting Strategies Fail

As the days turned into weeks and weeks turned into months, each family realized that their usual parenting strategies were no longer effective. Michael and Sarah had always believed in the power of consistency—bedtimes, mealtimes, and clear rules were staples in their household. Yet these structures seemed to do little to prevent Liam's explosive reactions. Even positive reinforcement—which had worked well with their older children—appeared to have no impact on Liam. He would earn a sticker for good behavior one moment, only to tear it up in frustration the next.

Raj and Priya had tried reasoning with Anika, appealing to her intelligence and usually calm nature. They had always been able to talk things through with her before, but now their words seemed to bounce off a wall of anger and sadness they couldn't penetrate. They tried giving her space, but that only seemed to intensify her feelings of isolation and despair. She became increasingly irritable. Everyone in the family felt as if they were walking on eggshells around her.

The shift in their environment and consequently their parenting style was tough for David and Elena. They had always been a laid-back, go-with-the-flow kind of family and had encouraged their children to express themselves freely, but given Maya's increasing volatility, they found themselves constantly on alert for the next outburst. Their once-harmonious home had become a place of tension and unpredictability.

In each household, the realization dawned slowly but unmistakably: this was more than just a phase, more than typical childhood moodiness. The strategies that had worked for their other children and that they had always relied upon as parents were failing them now. Each family also began to feel a deepening sense of isolation, assuming that they were the only ones struggling with such intense and frequent emotional storms. They were desperate for a solution, but where could they turn?

Recognizing When Something Is Wrong

The parents' journey toward understanding began with a nagging sense that something was fundamentally different about their child's emotional responses. For Michael and Sarah, it was the way Liam's irritability seemed to linger long after his initial outburst had subsided. Even in moments of calm, he had an undercurrent of tension, a readiness to explode at the slightest provocation. His teachers began to notice it, too, mentioning that Liam was easily frustrated at school, unable to tolerate even minor setbacks without becoming visibly upset.

Raj and Priya started to see a similar pattern in Anika. What had used to be isolated incidents of frustration were now daily occurrences, and the intensity of her reactions was far beyond what they had ever expected from her. It wasn't just about the outbursts, it was how her mood seemed to hover on the edge of anger or sadness, rarely dipping into happiness or contentment. The usual joys of childhood seemed to have lost their appeal for her, replaced by a constant irritability that was affecting her relationships with friends and family.

For David and Elena, Maya's change was equally heartbreaking—their once joyful daughter was now prone to fits of anger that seemed to come out of nowhere, leaving her exhausted and tearful. Maya's teachers reported that she struggled to concentrate in class, often withdrawing from group activities she had previously loved. The bright, eager child they all knew was slipping away, replaced by a girl they barely recognized.

These realizations were challenging to confront, but they were the parents' first step toward understanding that their children might be dealing with something beyond the ordinary challenges of growing up. The families began to research and talk to friends; eventually, they reached out to professionals. They learned that they were not alone—other parents were facing similar challenges, and there was a name for what their children might be experiencing: Disruptive Mood Dysregulation Disorder, or DMDD.

The Emotional Toll on Families

The emotional toll on these three families was immense. Michael and Sarah often argued about how they should handle Liam's behavior, and their frustration over him spilled into their relationship with each other. They were exhausted from the outbursts and the constant worry that they were somehow failing their son. Every day felt like a battle; they couldn't remember the last time they had enjoyed a peaceful moment as a family.

> My son's behavior caused immense strains on relationships with those around us. My mother told me he looked possessed when he was in a rage and that I needed to have him exorcised. My sister uninvited us from her wedding, claiming he would ruin it. We were never invited to family events or holidays, as he was viewed as being intentionally out of control. I was constantly told that I needed to put him in an institution. He didn't have friends at school since his behavior was so violent, and no one wanted him around. Our world has become so small. The judgment from strangers was one thing, but hurtful words from family were the worst.

Raj and Priya were likewise dealing with their own sense of loss. The calm, joyful daughter they had known seemed to have disappeared, replaced by a child they didn't understand. They missed the easy conversations they'd formerly had with Anika; they missed the laughter that had once filled their home. Now even the most straightforward interactions would become tense as Raj and Priya tried to navigate their daughter's unpredictable moods.

For David and Elena, the changes in Maya's behavior were a source of deep sorrow. They mourned the loss of their easygoing, happy child and struggled with guilt—had they done something wrong? Their once-vibrant home had become a place of stress and anxiety, where every day felt like a test of their patience and resilience.

These families weren't just attempting to manage their children's behavior, they were also grappling with the emotional fallout of it. The constant stress was taking a toll on their relationships, their mental health, and their overall sense of well-being. They felt isolated— surely no one else could understand what they were going through.

The First Steps to Seeking Help

When families face these situations, acknowledging the problem is often the hardest step for parents, especially when it comes to evaluating their child's emotional and behavioral wellbeing. For the families of Liam, Anika, and Maya, it took years of intense struggles, sleepless nights, and a gnawing sense of helplessness before they could fully admit to themselves that something was fundamentally different about their child's emotional responses. This realization wasn't just about recognizing that their usual parenting techniques were ineffective, it was also about facing the possibility that their child was dealing with something far beyond the typical challenges of childhood.

For Michael and Sarah, the moment of acknowledgment came during a particularly intense outburst from Liam that left them both physically and emotionally drained. They had exhausted every strategy they knew, from setting clear boundaries to offering comfort, but nothing seemed to reach their son. As they sat together in the quiet aftermath of the storm, they looked at each other and almost wordlessly understood that they needed help. It wasn't about their capabilities as parents, it was about understanding that Liam's struggles required more than they could provide on their own.

Raj and Priya faced a similar reckoning after one of Anika's most severe meltdowns. They had always prided themselves on their ability to communicate with their daughter, to guide her through her emotions with love and logic. But as Anika's outbursts became more frequent and intense, they began to see that their usual approaches were failing. The realization came with a mix of grief and relief—grief for the daughter they felt they were losing to anger and sadness and relief in understanding that seeking professional help was not a sign of failure but of love and commitment to her well-being.

For David and Elena, the turning point was the impact of Maya's behavior on their entire family dynamic. What began as occasional tantrums had escalated into daily battles, leaving everyone on edge. Before, their home had been filled with laughter and warmth, but now it was a place of tension and unpredictability. The breaking point came when David snapped at Maya in frustration, something he had never done before. The guilt and sadness that followed made it clear to both him and Elena that they needed to reach out for support, not just for Maya, but for the sake of their entire family.

> As a father of two children with DMDD, I am always observing any possible triggers that effect my children's mood and outbursts. I noticed that when my son played video games on a small device, like his handheld console, he would become more irritable, and outbursts were more likely to happen. There was a notable difference from when he played the same video games but on a larger device, like his desktop or television screen. I dug into research and found out that the seconds per frame were different between the screen sizes and concluded that the small devices may stimulate the brain activity differently, resulting in dysregulation. I also noticed similar reactions to strobe lights and seizure-prone games, particularly those that display warnings in arcades, had a similar effect.

Finally, each family reached a point where they knew they couldn't do it alone. The Browns were the first to consult their pediatrician, who referred them to a child psychologist who specialized in mood disorders. The Guptas reached out to a family therapist whom a friend had recommended. The Morgans—after many sleepless nights and long discussions—decided to seek help from a child psychiatrist.

Seeking help was the next critical step for these families. Doing so required them to move past the fear of judgment and the stigma that still surrounds mental health challenges, especially when those challenges are happening to children. Each family had their reservations—worries about what a diagnosis might mean, concerns about the impact of therapy or medication, the implications for their child's future—but they knew that continuing to struggle alone was not an option.

In their first meetings with professionals, the families began to learn about DMDD. They heard terms like "emotional dysregulation" and "mood disorders." They started to understand that their children's behavior was not a result of poor parenting or a lack of discipline. It was something deeper that needed to be understood and managed with the right tools and support.

The professionals they met with offered initial assessments and began to outline possible treatment plans. While the road ahead seemed daunting, there was also relief—finally, there was a name for what their children were experiencing! With that name came the possibility of finding ways to help them.

A new world of understanding emerged. The families learned about Disruptive Mood Dysregulation Disorder (DMDD), a recent addition to the childhood diagnostic system. The parents began to see that their child's behavior was the result of a complex neurological condition that needed specific care and attention. This knowledge brought a mix of emotions: sadness for the challenges their children would face and a sense of hope that things could get better with the proper support.

Understanding DMDD came in stages—it was a gradual process alternately filled with moments of clarity, confusion, hope, and doubt. However, with each new piece of information and each discussion with a therapist or doctor, the families felt a little better equipped to help their children. They learned to see their children's outbursts not as willful disobedience but as symptoms of a disorder that could be managed with the right strategies. While their journey ahead would be challenging, it would also be filled with potential for growth and healing.

As the families of Liam, Anika, and Maya began to navigate this new terrain, they found solace in knowing they weren't alone. They connected with other parents facing similar challenges and found strength in shared experiences and mutual support. The path ahead was still daunting, but they no longer faced it in isolation.

In the end, these first steps—acknowledging the problem, seeking help, and beginning to understand DMDD—marked the beginning of each family's journey toward resilience and empowerment. It was the start of a new chapter in their lives, one in which they could approach their child's needs with compassion, patience, and hope, knowing that they were not alone and that there were paths forward that could lead to a brighter future for their family.

Raising Resilient Children with DMDD

Raising a child with DMDD requires a thoughtful, compassionate, and structured approach. In this book, we introduce eight fundamental principles or "guideposts" designed to help parents foster emotional resilience in children who have DMDD. Bob and Sam have developed and written about these guideposts in many of their past books, including *Raising Resilient Children, Nurturing Resilience in Our Children,* and *Raising Resilient Children with Autism Spectrum Disorders.* These guideposts offer practical strategies that—when applied consistently!—create a supportive home environment where children with DMDD can thrive despite their challenges. Each guidepost targets a specific aspect of emotional resilience; in all, these guideposts provide a comprehensive approach to supporting children who have DMDD.

Raising a resilient child with DMDD requires a structured approach grounded in empathy, effective communication, and positive reinforcement. While we've devoted a chapter in this book to each of the guideposts, first we'll provide an overview of them here. These eight guideposts provide a comprehensive framework that parents can use to support a child's emotional and behavioral growth while fostering a supportive and nurturing environment.

1. **Teaching and conveying empathy:** Empathy is the cornerstone of emotional resilience. To cultivate empathy in their child, parents must first model it in daily interactions, including actively listening to a child, acknowledging their feelings, and showing compassion. By demonstrating empathy, we teach children to understand and relate to the emotions of others. Creating opportunities for a child to practice empathy—whether by helping others, caring for pets, or engaging in community service—reinforces this essential skill. Discussing emotions openly helps children recognize and label their feelings, which is crucial for developing empathy.
2. **Effective communication and listening actively:** Communication is critical in building a strong, supportive relationship with a child. Listening without judgment and validating a child's emotions create a safe space for them to express themselves. When parents respond with understanding and empathy, they foster trust and openness. Practical strategies such as maintaining eye contact, using affirmative gestures, and encouraging verbal cues enhance active listening. Mastering these communication skills helps a child feel heard and valued, ultimately contributing to their emotional stability.
3. **Accepting children for who they are:** Unconditional love and acceptance are powerful tools for a child's development, especially with respect to children with DMDD—they often struggle with intense emotions, and knowing they are loved despite these challenges reassures them. Demonstrating unconditional love through consistent support and affection helps a child build a strong sense of self-worth. Additionally, setting realistic expectations that align with a child's unique abilities prevents frustration and promotes confidence. Celebrating a

child's strengths, no matter how small, reinforces their self-esteem and strengthens their resilience.
4. **Nurturing "islands of competence":** Identifying and nurturing a child's strengths, or "islands of competence," is vital in boosting their confidence. Every child has unique talents, and focusing on these areas allows a child to excel and develop a positive self-image. Parents can encourage exploration and growth by providing resources for their children, enrolling them in classes, and/or connecting them with mentors who can help them build on their strengths. Setting achievable goals that align with a child's abilities fosters a sense of accomplishment and reduces feelings of frustration and failure.
5. **Helping children learn from rather than feel defeated by mistakes:** Teaching a child to view mistakes as learning opportunities rather than failures is crucial for building resilience. By fostering a growth mindset, parents help their child develop perseverance. Parents can model this mindset in daily interactions with their child by sharing their experiences with their own mistakes and how they learned from them. Through reflective questioning, parents can help their child analyze their actions and develop problem-solving skills. Parents can also emphasize the importance of effort over innate ability to encourage their children to persist despite any difficulties they may be having.
6. **Teaching children to solve problems and make sound decisions:** Problem-solving and decision-making are essential skills for fostering independence and confidence. A child can be taught to approach problems systematically when parents provide a structured framework for doing so. Within that kind of setting, a child can learn to identify problems, generate potential solutions, and evaluate the pros and cons of each option. When parents implement and monitor the chosen solution, they help their child learn from the outcome and build resilience through reflecting on what happened. Consistently applying this framework empowers a child to navigate through challenges with greater confidence.
7. **Disciplining in ways that promote self-discipline and self-worth:** Effective discipline rather than discipline rooted in punitive measures fosters self-discipline and selfworth, and positive reinforcement plays a crucial role in encouraging desirable behaviors. A child can be taught to understand expectations and feel good about meeting them when parents consistently recognize and reward positive actions. Maintaining consistent rules and expectations provides security and structure for all children! It's particularly important to create that kind of atmosphere for children with DMDD. Understanding the underlying reasons for a child's behavior and applying empathetic discipline helps the child manage their emotions more effectively.
8. **Developing responsibility, compassion, and a social conscience:** Teaching responsibility, compassion, and social conscience helps a child understand the impacts of their actions on others. Parents can encourage their child to take responsibility for their behavior through real-life examples and engaging activities. Cultivating empathy and emotional intelligence allows a child to connect with others and recognize their feelings. An example of this is involving children

in community service and social justice education—both foster a sense of social responsibility and empower children to contribute positively to society.

These eight guideposts provide a framework for parents to raise emotionally resilient children with DMDD. By consistently applying these principles even when challenged by a child's emotional turmoil, parents create a nurturing environment that empowers their child to navigate the complexities of DMDD with confidence and stability. This comprehensive approach supports the child's emotional development, strengthens the entire family, and lays the foundation for a future filled with hope and resilience.

Final Words

Three children in three families, each struggling with the unpredictable and often overwhelming manifestations of DMDD. Liam, Anika, and Maya's challenges went beyond typical childhood tantrums or mood swings—their reactions were intense, frequent, and seemingly out of their control, leaving their families in a state of perpetual anxiety and confusion. The Browns, Guptas, and Morgans shared a journey marked by a relentless quest for answers. They each sought the help of professionals, hoping to find a way to help their children. Through consultations with pediatricians, therapists, and specialists, they came to understand that their children were not merely "difficult" or "spoiled" but were grappling with a genuine neurological disorder.

For parents embarking on the daunting journey of raising a child with DMDD, the voyage often seems shrouded in a mist of uncertainty and isolation. The unpredictable nature of DMDD can leave families feeling adrift in a sea of confusion, struggling to navigate the choppy waters of intense emotional outbursts and persistent irritability that characterize the disorder. The sense of helplessness and isolation that parents often experience can be overwhelming, yet it's crucial for them to remember that they are not alone in navigating these waters.

This book is designed to be a lighthouse in the fog—we want to guide parents through the complexities of DMDD. In these pages, we delve deep into this disorder's origins, nuances, and intricacies, aiming to illuminate the path ahead with knowledge and understanding. By dispelling myths and misconceptions about DMDD, we strive to help parents and their children chart a course toward resilience and empowerment.

In the following chapters, we provide insights into the latest research and treatment strategies for DMDD: from cognitive-behavioral therapy (CBT) to medication, from parent training programs to educational interventions, we explore a range of practical approaches to managing the symptoms of DMDD. These treatments are not one-size-fits-all solutions; instead, they can be tailored to fit the unique needs of a child and their family. All of these treatments and interventions are built on the eight guideposts so that parents can raise resilient children regardless of their challenges.

In addition to professional interventions, we emphasize the importance of building a supportive community. This can include connecting with other families who are facing similar challenges, joining support groups, and/or engaging in family therapy. These connections can provide a sense of solidarity, reduce feelings of isolation, and offer practical advice and emotional support.

We'll also be addressing the impact of DMDD on siblings and the entire family. Siblings may feel neglected or overwhelmed by the intense focus on the child with DMDD, for example, and it's not unusual for both parents and siblings to experience PTSD symptoms from living in constant uncertainty and chaos. We discuss strategies to ensure that siblings feel valued and supported and we describe ways to maintain a balanced family dynamic.

Education plays a crucial role in the life of a child with DMDD! We'll explore the ways in which parents can work effectively with schools and educators to ensure that their child receives the appropriate accommodations and support. This includes advocating for their child's needs, understanding their educational rights, and fostering a collaborative relationship with teachers and school administrators.

As we chart this course together, it's essential to celebrate small victories and recognize a child's progress. Each step forward—no matter how incremental—is a testament to a parent's dedication and love. This journey is not just about managing a disorder, it's about parents understanding their child, fostering their strengths, and helping them realize their full potential.

A word about the families in this book: the Brown, Gupta, and Morgan families represent composites of the children we have worked with in our clinical practices. When we tally our combined experiences in this field, together, we have nearly 100 years of working with challenging children. The stories that begin and end each of the following chapters present real children and their families that our co-authors Donna and Molly compiled for our clinical textbook on DMDD (*Clinician Guide to Disruptive Mood Dysregulation Disorder in Children and Adolescents*).

In conclusion, this book is more than just a guide, it's a companion for parents to use during their journey of raising a child with DMDD. It's a source of knowledge, a tool for empowerment, and a beacon of hope. We hope parents gain insights and strategies to help light the way forward as they turn each page. Remember, knowledge is power—the power to understand, support, and guide a child toward a brighter, more resilient future.

Chapter 2
Understanding DMDD

Ben's Story

As Jennifer Bergen was sitting at her son Ben's high school graduation in their small rural Idaho town, an intense wave of emotion rushed over her when she heard his name announced. Overwhelmed with a mix of emotions, Jennifer wondered, "How did we get to graduation day?" While Ben walked across the stage to be handed his diploma, Jennifer thought back to just five years ago, when she had been about to reluctantly hand Ben over as a ward of the state knowing that he would have been permanently institutionalized in a psychiatric facility. The thought of that still made her shudder.

That horrid day was forever etched into her memory. That was the day when Ben, then 12 years old, had raged for hours and had landed in the pediatric ward of a psychiatric hospital nearly seven hours away from their home. It was the only facility with an available bed. That had been Ben's third psychiatric hospitalization, but this one had changed the course of his life.

Ben had had a particularly violent episode and had been placed in the seclusion room, where a team of 12 adults had struggled to restrain him so a doctor could sedate him with a powerful tranquilizer. That day, Jennifer had made the heartbreaking decision to sign custody of her son over to the state of Idaho. "I numbly filled out the paperwork and submitted it," she said later. "I dove head-first into a deep depression—I wouldn't be able to see my son's beautiful face every morning. I wouldn't get to give Ben squeezes or hugs when he needed some reassurance. I felt like I had failed as a parent—I knew that my son would grow up within the walls of a hospital with a nurse tending to him."

Up until that point, Jennifer had tried everything she'd been advised to do to help her middle child while attempting to keep Ben's two siblings and herself safe during the violent rages that would strike without warning. For years, the interventions she'd used with Ben had included alternative treatments, dietary changes, dozens of medications, and seemingly endless evaluations. He also received occupational therapy, counseling, and community-based rehabilitation.

Jennifer thought back to that time. "We were passed from clinic to clinic, with doctors telling me there was nothing they could do for him because nothing they had tried had helped," she remembered. "At age 10, Ben went through yet another battery of tests. Then DMDD and depression were added to his collection of diagnoses, a list that included ADHD, PTSD, and anxiety. During all of this, I was attending college and received my degrees in sociology and psychology. I studied those subjects out of desperation—I couldn't find anyone who could figure out what was driving my son's behavior or how to mitigate it other than keeping him sedated."

We'll return to Ben's story later, after we've comprehensively explored DMDD, focusing on its symptoms, diagnostic criteria, contributing factors, developmental roots, and treatment. DMDD is a condition characterized by severe temper outbursts and chronic irritability that affects children and adolescents. This chapter offers a foundational understanding of DMDD for parents, caregivers, and mental health professionals.

Overview and Symptoms of DMDD

DMDD is a relatively new diagnosis in the field of child and adolescent psychiatry. It was first introduced in the *Diagnostic and Statistical Manual of the American Psychiatric Association (DSM-5)* in 2013 and adopted a few years later by the International Classification of Diseases (ICD-11). The diagnosis was developed in response to the need for a category that could accurately describe and define children who exhibit severe irritability and frequent temper outbursts but do not fit the criteria for bipolar disorder or other mood disorders. DMDD is characterized by a persistent pattern of severe irritability and anger, with frequent temper outbursts that are grossly out of proportion to the situation. These symptoms are chronic, not episodic, and must be present for at least one year for a child to meet the diagnostic criteria.

Children with DMDD often experience intense emotional reactions to minor provocations, leading to outbursts that can include verbal rages or physical aggression. Unlike typical mood swings, the irritability in DMDD is pervasive and occurs most of the day, nearly every day. This persistent irritability is observable by others (parents, teachers, peers) and it significantly impairs the child's ability to function in daily life. The outbursts and irritability associated with DMDD are more severe than what's typically seen in children with other mood disorders, making the condition particularly challenging for affected families.

Early identification and intervention are crucial in managing DMDD effectively. Recognizing the signs of DMDD early can lead to more timely and appropriate interventions, which may improve outcomes for the child. Parents and caregivers play a vital role in identifying these symptoms, as they're often the first to notice the intense and frequent emotional outbursts that disrupt the child's daily functioning.

Understanding the symptoms of DMDD can also help differentiate it from other disorders with overlapping features, such as oppositional defiant disorder (ODD) and Attention-Deficit/Hyperactivity Disorder (ADHD).

The impact of DMDD extends beyond the child to the rest of the family because the frequent outbursts and pervasive irritability can strain family relationships and create a chaotic home environment. Parents may struggle with frustration, helplessness, and guilt as they manage their child's behavior. Siblings may also be affected—they may experience anxiety or resentment due to the constant tension and disruptions at home. Therefore, understanding DMDD is essential for recognizing and treating the disorder in a child and supporting the entire family.

Diagnostic Criteria for DMDD

The Diagnostic and Statistical Manual of Mental Disorders, Fifth Edition Text Revision (DSM-5-TR) provides specific criteria for diagnosing DMDD in children. These criteria are designed to ensure that the diagnosis is accurate and that another mental health condition does not better explain the symptoms. To receive a diagnosis of DMDD, a child must consistently exhibit the following symptoms over a specified period and in multiple settings:

Recurrent and Severe Temper Tantrums or Outbursts

The hallmark of DMDD is temper outbursts disproportionate to the situation or provocation. These outbursts can be verbal or behavioral, such as yelling, screaming, hitting, or throwing objects. The intensity and frequency of these outbursts are far beyond what would be expected for the child's developmental level. The *DSM-5* specifies that these outbursts must occur on average three or more times per week.

Persistent Irritability or Anger

In addition to temper outbursts, children with DMDD exhibit a persistently irritable or angry mood most of the day, nearly every day. This mood is observable by others (parents, teachers, peers) and is not confined to specific situations. The pervasive irritability or anger affects the child's interactions across different environments and relationships.

Duration of Symptoms

For a diagnosis of DMDD, its symptoms must be present for at least 12 months. During this period, the child must not have experienced a symptom-free interval lasting longer than three consecutive months. This criterion ensures that the mood disturbance is chronic and does not result from a temporary stressor or an adjustment period.

Onset of Symptoms

While the DSM criteria for DMDD don't address the timing or rate of symptom onset, it's worth mentioning that symptoms shouldn't appear suddenly, as that could indicate PANS (Pediatric Acute-onset Neuropsychiatric Syndrome) or PANDAS (Pediatric Autoimmune Neuropsychiatric Disorders Associated with Streptococcal Infections).

PANS and PANDAS are conditions where children experience a rapid onset of neuropsychiatric symptoms, such as OCD (obsessive-compulsive disorder), tics, and emotional dysregulation. Those are often triggered by infections or immune responses. PANDAS occurs explicitly after a streptococcal infection, while various infections or environmental factors can trigger PANS. These syndromes can mimic DMDD and lead to misdiagnosis. Several parents have reported cases where their children were initially diagnosed with DMDD but were later found to have PANS or PANDAS. Once treated for these conditions, their DMDD-like symptoms improved significantly. However, in cases where diagnosis and treatment were delayed, the neurological damage became more challenging to reverse.

The distinction between PANS or PANDAS and DMDD is crucial because the majority of children with DMDD do not experience a "rapid onset" of symptoms. Therefore, the appearance of sudden, severe behavioral changes could warrant further investigation into PANS or PANDAS. Recognizing the correct condition could help ensure timely and appropriate treatment, potentially preventing long-term damage. As of the time of this writing, there isn't any research demonstrating that children with PANS or PANDAS benefit from the medication treatments that benefit many youth with DMDD.

Settings

DMDD symptoms must be present in at least two primary settings: home, school, or social. Furthermore, the symptoms must be severe in at least one of these settings. This criterion is crucial in distinguishing DMDD from other conditions, as it highlights the disorder's pervasive nature across different areas of the child's life.

Age of Onset

DMDD should not be diagnosed before age six or after age 18; the onset of symptoms occurs before the age of 10. This criterion recognizes that irritability and temper outbursts are expected in early childhood but should decrease as children mature. Persistent and severe irritability that extends into middle childhood and adolescence is indicative of DMDD.

Exclusion of Other Disorders

Before diagnosing DMDD, clinicians must rule out other mental health conditions that could explain the child's symptoms, such as major depressive disorder, bipolar disorder, posttraumatic stress disorder (PTSD), or autism spectrum disorder. DMDD cannot be diagnosed if the symptoms occur exclusively during a major depressive episode or are better accounted for by another disorder.

The *DSM-5-TR* criteria for DMDD are designed to ensure that the diagnosis is specific and accurately reflects the severity and chronicity of the child's mood disturbance. Proper diagnosis is essential for guiding treatment, as DMDD requires a different approach than other mood disorders or behavioral issues. By adhering to these criteria, clinicians can more effectively identify children with DMDD and develop appropriate interventions to address their unique needs.

The Developmental Roots of DMDD

The developmental roots of DMDD are deeply intertwined with early childhood experiences and temperament—research has shown that children with certain temperamental traits and early developmental challenges are more prone to developing DMDD. Understanding these developmental roots is critical for identifying at-risk children and implementing early interventions to prevent the disorder from taking hold.

Temperament refers to the innate personality traits that influence how children respond to their environment. It's generally stable across a person's lifespan and becomes evident early in infancy. Children with a "difficult" temperament characterized by high reactivity, low adaptability, and poor self-regulation are at higher risk of developing DMDD. High reactivity means these children are likelier to have intense emotional responses to stimuli that evoke frustration or disappointment. They may cry more frequently, exhibit extreme expressions of joy or distress, and have difficulty calming down after becoming upset. This high reactivity can lead to frequent temper outbursts and persistent irritability, which are hallmark symptoms of DMDD.

DMDD is classified as a depressive disorder, meaning that children with DMDD may exhibit not only irritability but also feelings of helplessness and hopelessness. This can manifest as sadness or depressive behaviors in addition to irritability. Children with DMDD can appear sad or depressed, as these emotions often co-occur with irritability. A child's sadness and irritability may reflect the broader emotional experience that's common in children with DMDD.

Low adaptability is another temperamental trait associated with DMDD. Children with low adaptability have difficulty adjusting to new situations or changes in routine. They may become easily overwhelmed by transitions, unexpected events, cancellations, or plans not meeting their expectations, all of which lead to increased stress and irritability. For example, a child with low adaptability may struggle with changes in their daily schedule, such as starting a new school year, moving to a new home, or having events be canceled. Again, all of those can trigger emotional outbursts and exacerbate symptoms of DMDD.

Early Childhood Development

The early developmental period is a critical time for forming self-regulation skills essential for managing emotions and behaviors. Self-regulation involves controlling one's emotional responses, delaying gratification, and maintaining focus in the face of distractions. Children who struggle with self-regulation are more likely to develop DMDD, as they may have difficulty managing their emotions and impulses. Early disruptions in attachment, such as inconsistent caregiving or emotional neglect, can further impair the development of selfregulation skills and contribute to the onset of DMDD.

Attachment theory posits that a child's early experiences with caregivers is crucial to their emotional development. Secure attachment—characterized by consistent and responsive caregiving—provides a foundation for healthy emotional regulation. In contrast, *in*secure attachment that results from inconsistent or neglectful caregiving can lead to emotional dysregulation and an increased risk of developing DMDD. Children who experience insecure attachment may have difficulty trusting others, regulating their emotions, and forming healthy relationships, all of which can contribute to the development of DMDD.

The interplay between temperament and early childhood experiences creates a developmental trajectory that can lead to the onset of DMDD. Children with a problematic temperament who also experience early disruptions in attachment and self-regulation are particularly vulnerable to developing the disorder. Understanding these developmental roots allows for early identification of at-risk children and the implementation of preventive interventions, such as parent training programs and early childhood mental health services, which can help mitigate the risk of DMDD and promote healthy emotional development.

Contributing Factors to DMDD

A complex interplay of genetic, neurobiological, and environmental factors influences the development of DMDD. Understanding these contributing factors is crucial for developing effective prevention and treatment strategies. While research on DMDD is still evolving, several key factors have been identified that contribute to the disorder's onset and progression.

Genetic Factors

There's evidence to suggest that DMDD has a genetic component, with specific genes related to emotional regulation and impulsivity potentially playing a role. Family and twin studies have shown that children with DMDD are more likely to have relatives with mood disorders, suggesting a hereditary link. For example, polymorphisms (the occurrence of two or more different alleles or genetic variants at a particular gene locus within a population that leads to different traits or phenotypes) in serotonin-related (neurotransmitter) genes, which are involved in mood regulation, have been associated with an increased risk of developing DMDD. Additionally, genes related to the neurotransmitters dopamine and norepinephrine pathways, which are implicated in impulsivity and aggression, may also contribute to the disorder. However, the genetic basis of DMDD is complex and not fully understood, and further research is needed to clarify the specific genetic mechanisms involved.

Neurobiological Factors

Neurobiological abnormalities are believed to underlie the emotional dysregulation observed in DMDD. Neuroimaging studies have shown that children with DMDD often exhibit differences in brain structure and function, particularly in areas involved in emotion regulation, such as the prefrontal cortex and amygdala. The prefrontal cortex, responsible for decisionmaking, impulse control, and emotional regulation, may be less active or less developed in children with DMDD. Similarly, the amygdala, which processes emotional stimuli and triggers emotional responses, may be hyperactive in these children, leading to heightened emotional reactivity and frequent outbursts.

Additionally, abnormalities in the connectivity between the prefrontal cortex and the amygdala have been observed. This disrupted communication may impair the child's ability to regulate emotional responses, contributing to the intense irritability and anger outbursts characteristic of DMDD. Functional connectivity deficits between these brain regions hinder the ability to modulate emotional experiences effectively, leading to heightened emotional responses in situations that might otherwise be managed with more controlled reactions.

Dysregulation of neurotransmitters like serotonin and dopamine also plays a role in the development of DMDD. Low levels of serotonin are often associated with irritability and aggression, both core symptoms of DMDD. Dopamine, a neurotransmitter associated with reward processing, may also be dysregulated in children with DMDD, leading to difficulties in processing and responding appropriately to rewards and frustrations. This imbalance can exacerbate mood instability, frustration tolerance, and aggressive behavior.

Environmental Factors

Environmental factors significantly contribute to developing and maintaining DMDD symptoms. Adverse experiences such as chronic stress, trauma, neglect, or inconsistent parenting can disrupt a child's emotional development and contribute to the dysregulation of emotions. For example, children who are exposed to high levels of family conflict, harsh discipline, or parental psychopathology are at increased risk of developing DMDD. These environmental stressors can exacerbate the child's existing vulnerabilities (i.e., a problematic temperament or genetic predisposition) and lead to the development of severe mood dysregulation. On the other hand, positive environmental factors like supportive parenting, stable family relationships, and access to mental health resources can help mitigate the impact of these stressors and reduce the risk of DMDD.

Similar to many childhood emotional disorders, the symptoms of DMDD can be exacerbated by various environmental and lifestyle factors: poor diet, limited sleep, and chaotic home life can all contribute to the worsening of DMDD behaviors. A child's emotional regulation is often sensitive to these stressors, which can intensify irritability and temper outbursts. In families facing multiple risk factors (socioeconomic challenges, instability at home, etc.), these stressors may create an environment that makes it increasingly difficult for children to manage their emotions.

Some evidence suggests that poor nutrition and malnutrition can act as stressors that increase the risk of developing or exacerbating mental health issues, including mood disorders. Although specific research on the direct relationship between malnutrition and the development of DMDD is limited, there's broader scientific support for the role of diet in childhood emotional and behavioral disorders. For instance, deficiencies in essential nutrients like omega-3 fatty acids, zinc, and iron have been linked to increased aggression and mood dysregulation.

Low levels of vitamin D3 can also alter mood—some studies show a link between insufficient vitamin D3 and depression. That's because vitamin D3 deficiency can make it difficult for the body to produce serotonin, a hormone that stabilizes mood and increases happiness. Additionally, a diet high in processed foods, sugar, and unhealthy fats has been associated with negative impacts on mental health, particularly in children.

Given that children with DMDD already struggle to regulate their emotions, a poor diet can likely compound these difficulties, making symptoms more severe. Therefore, addressing dietary needs and ensuring proper nutrition could be critical to managing DMDD, especially in families dealing with multiple stressors. Ensuring that children have a balanced diet, adequate sleep, and a stable home environment may help reduce the severity of DMDD symptoms and improve overall emotional well-being.

Cumulative Impact

The interactions between genetic, neurobiological, and environmental factors create a cumulative impact that shapes the development and progression of DMDD. Over time, the combined effects of these factors can lead to a more severe and persistent pattern of emotional dysregulation. For example, a child with a genetic predisposition for emotional dysregulation who also experiences neurobiological abnormalities and significant environmental stressors is at a much higher risk of developing DMDD than a child who only has one of these risk factors. The cumulative impact of these factors can also influence the course of the disorder, with children who experience multiple risk factors being more likely to develop chronic and severe symptoms.

Timing and Developmental Milestones

The timing of these interactions is also critical. The early childhood and adolescent years are times of heightened vulnerability—the brain is still developing, and the effects of environmental stressors can have long-lasting consequences. Exposure to trauma or chronic stress during these critical periods can disrupt the development of emotional regulation skills and increase the risk of developing DMDD. How genetic, neurobiological, and environmental factors interact may vary depending on the child's developmental stage, with certain factors becoming more or less influential at different times.

Many parents (including those whose stories are shared in this book) seek help for their children long before an official diagnosis of DMDD is made. While the diagnosis typically happens around age six, beginning signs of emotional dysregulation often appear earlier. Our epidemiological research suggests that symptoms of DMDD can be reliably identified by age four, with patterns of irritability and emotional outbursts observable and reportable as early as age two. This early recognition is crucial, as families with children at risk for DMDD need not wait for a formal diagnosis to begin seeking support and intervention.

Understanding the interactions between genetic, neurobiological, and environmental factors is essential for developing effective prevention and treatment

> As a DMDD parent, we started addressing a range of issues that could be affecting our son's chronic irritability when he was a toddler. From the age of two to five, we treated him for allergies and asthma and addressed chronic inflammation with the removal of his adenoids and tonsils. We pursued therapies and medications to manage hyperactivity, insomnia, anxiety, and depression. He received his first Individualized Education Program (IEP) through the school district and started at the early intervention preschool. By the time he received the DMDD diagnosis, he was already accustomed to a routine of a structured classroom, taking medication, and seeing a therapist.

strategies for DMDD. By recognizing the complex interplay of these influences, clinicians can adopt a more holistic approach that addresses the root causes of the disorder. *Early intervention is key!* By addressing contributing factors *before* the disorder becomes entrenched, better outcomes are possible for children with DMDD. Be reassured, however, that parents do not cause DMDD.

Co-occurring Problems in DMDD

DMDD rarely exists in isolation—the disorder frequently co-occurs with other psychiatric conditions, complicating both diagnosis and treatment. This section delves into the common comorbidities associated with DMDD, highlighting the complex interplay between these disorders and the challenges they present in clinical settings.

ADHD and DMDD

One of the most prevalent co-occurring conditions with DMDD is Attention-Deficit/Hyperactivity Disorder (ADHD). Research indicates that a significant percentage of children diagnosed with DMDD also meet the criteria for ADHD, with estimates ranging from 25% to 45%. Both disorders share overlapping symptoms, such as impulsivity, emotional dysregulation, and behavioral challenges, making differential diagnoses particularly challenging. Many children initially diagnosed with ADHD are later found to have DMDD or other underlying mood disorders, complicating treatment approaches and outcomes.

A significant concern in these cases is the early prescription of stimulant medications, which are commonly used to manage ADHD symptoms. Although stimulants are effective in treating ADHD, they can magnify mood instability in children who also have undiagnosed mood disorders like DMDD. This can lead to a worsening of emotional dysregulation, increased irritability, and more extreme mood swings. For children with both ADHD and DMDD, stimulants may exacerbate their symptoms, particularly those related to mood instability, contributing to a more turbulent and challenging course of treatment.

Children with ADHD often exhibit difficulties with inattention, hyperactivity, and impulsivity. When ADHD co-occurs with DMDD, these symptoms are compounded by severe irritability and frequent temper outbursts, creating a more complex clinical picture. The presence of both disorders can exacerbate emotional dysregulation and lead to more intense behavioral issues and more significant impairment in social and academic settings. For instance, a child with both ADHD and DMDD may struggle not only with sustaining attention and controlling impulses but also with managing overwhelming emotions, resulting in frequent conflicts at school and home.

Parents and clinicians alike have raised concerns about the premature use of stimulants in young children, especially when ADHD is diagnosed before a thorough evaluation for mood disorders such as DMDD is conducted. Many parents have reported that their children were initially diagnosed with ADHD and treated with stimulants and then experienced severe mood deterioration and behavioral escalation, often before the correct diagnosis of DMDD was made. These adverse effects can manifest as increased aggression, emotional outbursts, anxiety, and even dangerous behaviors that may lead to crises, including hospitalization.

Additionally, ADHD is often the initial diagnosis given to children displaying symptoms like inattention, impulsivity, and hyperactivity—behaviors that are not uncommon in young children, particularly those at risk for mood and behavioral disorders. This overlap of symptoms frequently results in ADHD being identified first, as these behaviors are universally recognized while underlying mood disorders like DMDD may go unnoticed. Given that pediatricians and general practitioners are often the first to assess these children, stimulants are sometimes prescribed as early as age four or five. And because many pediatricians are only beginning to learn about DMDD through recent continuing education, DMDD may be underdiagnosed or the diagnosis might be delayed.

The result is that children who are later diagnosed with DMDD in addition to ADHD may endure months or even years of worsened symptoms due to stimulant treatment. This period can be especially difficult for children and their families, as the worsening of behaviors due to children being on stimulants can lead to severe emotional and behavioral challenges that impact not only the child's mental health but also the entire family's well-being. While a negative response to stimulants may eventually guide professionals toward a more appropriate diagnosis of DMDD, the process is often lengthy and stressful, with significant adverse effects experienced along the way.

Parent reports have consistently highlighted the difficulty of managing children during this time. For many families, the worsening of symptoms under stimulant treatment was a pivotal reason why they advocated for further evaluation of their child, a process that ultimately led to a DMDD diagnosis. However, this period of misdiagnosis and inappropriate treatment can be highly distressing—some children even require hospitalization due to the severity of their behaviors. The frustration expressed by many parents points to the need for earlier recognition of mood disorders like DMDD and greater caution in prescribing stimulants for children who may have undiagnosed comorbidities.

Anxiety Disorders and DMDD

Anxiety disorders are another common comorbidity in children with DMDD. These disorders can include generalized anxiety disorder, separation anxiety, and social anxiety disorder. The chronic irritability and emotional instability inherent in DMDD can often fuel anxiety and vice versa. For example, a child with both DMDD and generalized anxiety disorder may experience heightened levels of worry and tension, which can trigger or exacerbate the explosive outbursts characteristic of DMDD. It's common for children with DMDD to exhibit avoidant behaviors such as repeatedly refusing to go to school. Many parents believe these behaviors are often linked to underlying anxiety. School refusal is a frequent concern reported by parents of children with DMDD, affecting children across various age groups.

The co-occurrence of anxiety disorders with DMDD can complicate effective treatment. Anxiety often requires interventions that focus on calming and reducing worry, whereas DMDD treatment may prioritize managing anger and irritability. Clinicians must carefully balance these approaches, ensuring that one set of symptoms is not inadvertently exacerbated while the other is being treated.

Oppositional Defiant Disorder (ODD) and DMDD

Oppositional Defiant Disorder (ODD) is another condition that's often diagnosed alongside DMDD. ODD is characterized by a persistent pattern of angry or irritable mood, argumentative or defiant behavior, and a tendency toward vindictiveness. Since both ODD and DMDD can involve irritability and frequent temper outbursts, it can be difficult for parents and professionals to tell the two conditions apart. However, the critical difference is that ODD primarily focuses on defiant and noncompliant behaviors, while DMDD is centered on mood dysregulation and extreme emotional reactions.

According to current diagnostic criteria, children with DMDD often exhibit behaviors similar to those seen in ODD. However, only about 15% of children diagnosed with ODD also meet the mood-related criteria necessary for a DMDD diagnosis. The *DSM* provides clear guidance in these cases: if a child meets the requirements for both DMDD and ODD, only the DMDD diagnosis should be given. DMDD is considered the more comprehensive diagnosis when mood dysregulation is the primary concern. This same rule applies if a child meets the criteria for both DMDD and intermittent explosive disorder—again, DMDD is the diagnosis that takes precedence.

For parents, it's helpful to focus more on overlapping symptoms than on labels. While irritability, defiance, and emotional outbursts may appear in both disorders, the real difference lies in whether mood instability or behavioral noncompliance is the more significant challenge for the child. If mood dysregulation is the primary issue, a DMDD diagnosis is likely more accurate. Understanding this distinction can help guide treatment decisions and ensure that the child receives the proper support for their emotional and behavioral needs.

When ODD and DMDD symptoms co-occur, a child may present with a combination of severe mood instability and defiant, oppositional behaviors. This combination often leads to significant difficulties in relationships with authority figures like parents and teachers. It can result in a higher likelihood of disciplinary actions in school as well as strained family dynamics.

Major Depression and DMDD

Major depression is also commonly seen in children with DMDD. The chronic irritability and negative mood associated with DMDD can be precursors to depressive disorders, particularly as the child moves into adolescence. Children with both DMDD and major depression may exhibit pervasive sadness, a lack of interest in activities, and feelings of hopelessness, alongside their irritability and temper outbursts.

The presence of major depression in a child with DMDD can lead to more adverse outcomes, including an increased risk of self-harm and suicidal ideation. Clinicians must monitor these children closely—particularly during stressful periods!—to provide timely interventions that address both the mood dysregulation of DMDD and the more persistent mood disturbances of depression.

Bipolar Disorder and DMDD

Bipolar disorder (BD) and DMDD are both characterized by mood disturbances. Still, they're distinct in their presentation and course. BD involves episodic mood changes, with clear periods of mania or hypomania (a less severe form of mania) alternating with depressive episodes. In contrast, DMDD is defined by chronic irritability and severe temper outbursts that occur frequently and are not limited to distinct episodes. Unlike BD, DMDD does *not* include the elevated or expansive mood seen in mania. The distinction is crucial for diagnosis and treatment, as misdiagnosing a child with BD when they actually have DMDD can lead to inappropriate treatment strategies. Understanding these differences helps clinicians provide more accurate diagnoses and tailored interventions, ensuring that children receive the most effective care for their conditions. This understanding is vital for both parents and healthcare providers as they manage these complex and overlapping mood disorders.

Unfortunately, some mental health professionals may insist that DMDD is not a "real" diagnosis, often categorizing these children as having bipolar disorder. This misperception can lead to significant consequences in both diagnosis and treatment. Although both BD and DMDD involve mood disturbances, as previously noted, a critical difference exists: BD is characterized by distinct, episodic shifts between manic or hypomanic episodes and depression, while DMDD manifests as persistent irritability and frequent temper outbursts with*out* any episodic mood changes. When professionals dismiss DMDD as a valid diagnosis, they risk overdiagnosing

BD. That in turn can lead to inappropriate treatments, such as the use of mood stabilizers or antipsychotic medications that may not be suitable for children with DMDD.

This misdiagnosis can have long-term implications. Children with DMDD who are inaccurately diagnosed with BD may not receive specific behavioral interventions or therapeutic approaches that could more effectively address their chronic irritability and emotional regulation issues. As a result, these children might face unnecessary side effects from medications they don't need or they might miss out on evidence-based treatments tailored for DMDD. Clinicians absolutely must differentiate between the two disorders to provide appropriate care.

Intermittent Explosive Disorder and DMDD

Intermittent Explosive Disorder (IED) and DMDD both involve episodes of extreme anger and aggression, but they differ in crucial aspects. IED is characterized by sudden, impulsive outbursts of intense anger or aggression that are disproportionate to the situation and occur without a persistent irritable mood between episodes. These outbursts are typically brief and unplanned. In contrast, DMDD involves a more chronic pattern of severe irritability or angry mood between outbursts, along with frequent temper tantrums. It's important to note that according to diagnostic criteria, if a child presents symptoms that meet the requirements for both IED and DMDD, only the diagnosis of DMDD should be assigned. This ensures that the more persistent mood disturbance is appropriately recognized and treated.

While both disorders involve challenges with anger regulation, DMDD's ongoing irritability sets it apart from the more episodic nature of IED. Differentiating between these disorders is essential for accurate diagnosis and effective treatment, as the chronic mood dysregulation in DMDD requires a different therapeutic approach than the more episodic aggression seen in IED. Understanding these distinctions helps guide appropriate interventions and support for affected children and their families.

Autism Spectrum Disorder (ASD) and DMDD

Autism spectrum disorder (ASD) and DMDD can co-present in children, complicating the diagnostic process. Both conditions share overlapping symptoms, such as emotional outbursts, irritability, and difficulty managing frustration. However, the critical difference lies in the triggers and nature of these outbursts. Understanding this distinction is crucial for parents and professionals when determining the most accurate diagnosis and treatment plan.

Children with ASD often experience meltdowns in response to specific environmental triggers, such as changes in routine, sensory overload, or difficulty communicating their needs. These meltdowns are typically considered a direct consequence of their autism. The current diagnostic criteria emphasize that when a child with ASD exhibits temper outbursts in reaction to routine disruptions or sensory stimuli, these behaviors should be understood as part of the autism spectrum disorder rather than as a separate diagnosis of DMDD. In these cases, mood dysregulation is secondary to the underlying challenges associated with ASD, and DMDD would not be diagnosed.

In contrast, DMDD is characterized by chronic irritability and frequent, severe temper outbursts that occur without predictable external triggers. The emotional dysregulation in DMDD is pervasive, and children with this disorder often have difficulty controlling their emotions in a variety of settings regardless of specific disruptions or environmental changes.

When both ASD and DMDD are considered, professionals need to carefully evaluate the child's behavior within different contexts. If the emotional outbursts are primarily triggered by disruptions related to the child's autism, the diagnosis should focus on ASD. However, if the mood dysregulation appears to be more generalized and is not tied to autism-specific triggers, a separate diagnosis of DMDD may be appropriate.

Implications for Treatment of Co-occurring Conditions

The presence of co-occurring conditions in children with DMDD necessitates a comprehensive and individualized treatment approach, as the interplay between these disorders can significantly impact the overall therapeutic strategy. Each co-occurring disorder may require distinct therapeutic interventions, and the interactions between these conditions must be carefully considered. For instance, pharmacotherapy might be adjusted to simultaneously address ADHD symptoms and mood instability, ensuring that medications for one condition do not exacerbate the other; similarly, psychotherapy can be customized to tackle multiple issues concurrently, such as managing anxiety and anger or improving emotional regulation and social skills.

DMDD rarely exists in isolation, and the frequent co-occurrence of disorders such as ADHD, anxiety, Oppositional Defiant Disorder (ODD), and depression adds layers of complexity to both diagnosis and treatment. These overlapping conditions often share symptoms, making it challenging to differentiate between them, yet each requires targeted interventions. For example, a child with DMDD and anxiety may benefit from cognitive-behavioral therapy (CBT) that focuses on anxiety reduction techniques while also engaging in anger management strategies.

Understanding and addressing these comorbid conditions is crucial for developing effective, holistic treatment plans. A comprehensive approach improves the core symptoms of DMDD and enhances the overall functioning and quality of life for affected children and adolescents. This kind of holistic strategy can include a combination of medication, tailored psychotherapy, behavioral interventions, and family support, all aimed at addressing the unique needs of each child. Through this multifaceted approach, healthcare providers can create more effective and personalized treatment plans that lead to better long-term outcomes for children struggling with DMDD and its associated conditions.

Ben's Story Continues

Just days before Ben was to be transferred to the residential institution, Jennifer collected all of his records and started reading through years of treatments and observations. When she got to his testing result that said DMDD, she realized she had never investigated it since doctors had been telling her that his PTSD was driving his dysfunction.

Turning to the internet, Jennifer read research studies, blogs, and anything she could find on DMDD. "I couldn't believe what I had found—there were other families with kids like Ben!" she recalled. "Their stories were so similar to ours that I knew I had to dig deeper." Jennifer searched for medication interventions for DMDD and stumbled upon an article in *Psychiatric News* about a promising medication protocol.

Just then, Jennifer got the call that in three days, Ben would be transported to the institution. She needed to gather his belongings and say goodbye. The night before she left, she found lectures about DMDD given by Dr. Daniel Matthews and Dr. Larry Fisher on YouTube. "I saved the videos and listened to them while I started the seven-hour drive to my son. I listened intently to what the doctors said, and I yelled and cried as they talked about DMDD and its associated behaviors. They were talking about *Ben*, not just a diagnosis."

The next day, when Jennifer met with Ben's doctor and care team at the hospital, she tried to explain the research she had found and the promising protocol offered by Drs. Matthews and Fisher. Despite these new insights, however, the doctor still told her that it was time to give up. "He told me Ben was a danger to himself, his family, and society and needed to be locked into an institution and forgotten about," Jennifer said, traces of anger still in her voice. "I slammed my hand on the table and yelled, 'I haven't tried everything! I haven't tried *this*!' I removed Ben against medical advice, rescinded his application to the institution, and brought him home."

Several days later, with her new information in hand, Jennifer begged Ben's medication manager to start the Matthews Protocol. The doctor needed time to research the medication, but 10 days later, they started the protocol. That was the beginning of Ben's healing journey. "Four months later, my son was a completely different child," said Jennifer. "Ben went from being completely out of control to being a seemingly neurotypical child. The behavioral problems at school and home stopped. He was finally happy!"

Having the proper medication at the precise dosage Ben needed provided the foundation that became a launching pad for his future. Ben's athletic success led him to receive the prestigious "Captain of the Ship" basketball award during his junior year for team-building. His senior year, he was captain of the varsity basketball team. He then graduated from high school with a strong GPA and a scholarship to attend college for a future in welding.

But Ben's astounding progress wasn't due solely to pharmaceutical interventions—his mother, a Navy veteran, navigated the complexities of raising a child with DMDD with perseverance and tenacity. "I never lowered the bar for Ben," Jennifer said. "I have high expectations for all three of my children. I just parent Ben differently." Jennifer has provided and continues to provide a nurturing, consistent structure for her children, one that fosters emotional resilience, security, responsibility, and respect within her family unit and the greater community. She spent most of her parenting years as a single mother who never gave up on her child.

Implications for Treatment and Intervention

The complex interplay of genetic, neurobiological, and environmental factors in the development of DMDD has significant implications for treatment and intervention. Given the multifaceted nature of the disorder, a one-size-fits-all approach is unlikely to be effective. Instead, a comprehensive, multidimensional treatment strategy that addresses the various contributing factors is essential for effectively managing DMDD.

Pharmacotherapy

Given the neurobiological underpinnings of DMDD, pharmacotherapy is an essential component of the treatment plan for most affected children. Medications such as selective serotonin reuptake inhibitors (SSRIs) or mood stabilizers have been prescribed to address the dysregulation of neurotransmitters, particularly serotonin and dopamine (which are associated with mood and emotional regulation). However, the use of medication in children with DMDD is challenging. For one thing, children with DMDD may respond differently to these medications when compared with adults, so finding the correct dosage and combination of drugs can be a complex process. Moreover, the potential side effects of psychiatric medications—especially in young children—must be carefully weighed against the benefits.

> My daughter had been on almost three dozen different medications for seven years and was no better. During that time, she had been hospitalized three different times and was in a residential facility. It wasn't until I learned about Dr. Matthews Protocol from an online support group and found a doctor willing to try it that my daughter eventually got stable. I wish we had learned about this sooner, as it is the only thing that has helped stabilize her, bringing peace to our family.

The Matthews Protocol

The Matthews Protocol marks a notable shift in the treatment of DMDD for children and adolescents who struggle with extreme mood swings and aggressive behavior. Developed by Dr. Daniel Matthews, a pediatric neuropsychiatrist, the protocol offers a new approach that moves away from traditional reliance on antipsychotic medications and mood stabilizers, both of which often have limited effectiveness and significant side effects. Instead, Dr. Matthews has focused on the neurobiological origins of the disorder, utilizing a pharmacological strategy that has proven to be both safer and more effective.

Throughout his 40-plus-year career, Dr. Matthews concentrated on helping young patients with severe anger and impulsivity—now recognized as symptoms of DMDD. Unsatisfied with the results of conventional treatments and particularly the use of antipsychotics, Dr. Matthews explored alternative approaches. In the 1970s, his work led to the identification of abnormal brain activity in children with rage episodes. To achieve these observations, he used advanced tools like quantitative electroencephalograms (qEEG), a type of EEG that evokes the brain using audible and visual stimulation. Dr. Matthews identified an electrical abnormality in the brains of these children, who often had no recollection of their rage episodes. His findings suggested that the brain activity associated with outbursts in children with DMDD was similar to seizure-like brain activity, prompting a shift away from using antipsychotics and toward focusing on stabilizing the brain's neurobiology.

Building on these insights, Dr. Matthews found success in treating DMDD by using a combination of anticonvulsants like oxcarbazepine and the dopamine agonist called amantadine. He honed in on this combination during the time he spent managing an inpatient unit for aggressive children at Duke University, where he observed that many patients had no memory of their violent outbursts. Brain scans of these children showed overactivity in the amygdala, the brain's emotional center. This has been linked to low dopamine levels, which likely contributed to their heightened vigilance and lack of impulse control. These findings helped explain why stimulants—which enhance dopamine activity—appeared to alleviate symptoms in some cases. Matthews theorized that amantadine, a medicine that increases dopamine release and inhibits its reuptake, might be even more effective in reducing aggressive outbursts.

Clinical studies conducted by Dr. Matthews have demonstrated that this oxcarbazepine amantadine combination significantly reduces the chances of rehospitalization in children with severe irritability and recurrent outbursts. Furthermore, long-term tracking of patients treated with this regimen has shown that about 50% exhibit normalized amygdala activity as they move into adolescence, along with notable improvements in symptoms.

One possibility for the occurrence of these improvements is that over time, in some cases, new brain cells start to take on the appearance of calmer brain cells while patients are on this medication. In some instances, patients may need less medication and can slowly decrease or even discontinue it. Dr. Matthews also hypothesized that many children treated with this protocol required lower doses of medication as their brain stabilized. But in addition to this essential pharmacological treatment, Dr. Matthews also emphasized the importance of psychotherapy in helping these children recover. Many young patients have struggled with temper issues for most of their lives, he noted, and while medication can restore their chemical balance, they need behavioral therapy for their long-term rehabilitation.

The Matthews Protocol begins with administering oxcarbazepine, an anticonvulsant that also acts as a mood stabilizer (marketed as Trileptal® or Oxtellar®). Oxcarbazepine effectively addresses the seizure-like electrical abnormalities identified in Dr. Matthews' research, helping to stabilize mood and reduce the frequency of explosive outbursts. These factors are most effectively addressed with oxcarbazepine at a dosage of 35–50 mg/kg/day. Stability is typically achieved with a therapeutic blood level of 30–35. While titrating on oxcarbazepine, 150–300 mg increases every 7–10 days are suggested; however, most parents suggest only using 75–150 mg increases to avoid increased irritability during the titration period. Frequent blood labs are necessary to monitor levels and make dosage adjustments.

Common side effects of oxcarbazepine may include dizziness, fatigue, and the potential for a severe skin rash (Steven Johnson's Syndrome), particularly in individuals of Asian descent. Appropriate hydration in the form of fluids or tablets is necessary to offset any temporary side effects since anticonvulsants can deplete electrolyte and sodium levels in the body. Although numerous companies manufacture oxcarbazepine, it's best to stay with the same manufacturer— changing from one to another can alter the results.

Amantadine (marketed as Symmetrel® or Gocovri®) is typically added when a child is close to stability on the anticonvulsant medication. This antiviral and dopamine agonist (a type of drug that mimics the effects of dopamine by stimulating dopamine receptors in the brain, often used to treat conditions like Parkinson's disease or restless legs syndrome) has shown efficacy in supporting the frontal lobe and impacts impulsivity and executive functioning. Amantadine works by increasing dopamine and stimulating norepinephrine levels in the brain. This is crucial, because children with DMDD may require enhanced dopamine activity to effectively manage their symptoms. The maximum benefit dosage of amantadine is usually 200–400 mg daily, and the dosage is not based on blood levels but rather on behavior. It's best to increase by 50–100 mg weekly—little further benefit is seen beyond this dosage range. Dosages exceeding 15–20 mg/kg/day should be avoided due to the possibility of DNA damage in brain cells as well as the development of behavioral deficits that has been recently demonstrated at doses of 30–60 mg/kg/day (but were not evident in the 15 mg/kg/day dosage range).

Possible side effects of amantadine include decreased appetite, insomnia, constipation, and eye-related issues. In rare cases, psychosis can occur. In approximately 25% of children taking amantadine, the beneficial effect is lost between four and eight weeks; this is thought to be due to receptor exhaustion. This will be noticed by the sudden (not gradual) return of impulsive behavior and executive functioning. Should this occur, the medication should be stopped for 48 hours and then reintroduced at the previously effective dose—this is known as an amantadine break. It will likely be necessary to repeat these breaks for that same initial interval. If amantadine HCl alone does not provide sufficient benefit, then clonidine HCl can be added since the two do not have any drug/drug interactions and the HCl actions are at norepinephrine receptors. If the patient has had (or currently has) tics, then amantadine may rarely cause a reoccurrence or increase in tics due to amantadine's action at the D-1 and D-2 receptors. If this occurs, then the amantadine must be discontinued, at which point the tics should resolve. The combination of oxcarbazepine and amantadine will have effectively stabilized the brain's electrical activity, reducing extreme outbursts and the need for more invasive interventions like hospitalization.

The Matthews Protocol has demonstrated a consistent success rate of 85–90% in stabilizing children with DMDD in open-label trials. This is a significant improvement over traditional treatments! By addressing what Dr. Matthews believed was the root cause of the disorder—namely, electrical abnormalities in the brain—the protocol not only reduces the severity of symptoms but also decreases the need for multiple medication trials, which can be distressing for both the child and their family.

While the core of the Matthews Protocol involves oxcarbazepine and amantadine, Dr. Matthews recognized that not all patients will respond similarly to these medications. Alternative medications are considered for those who experience side effects or do not achieve the desired therapeutic outcomes—memantine, another NMDA receptor antagonist, can be substituted for amantadine; it offers a similar increase in dopamine activity with a different side effect profile.

Similarly, lamotrigine (Lamictal®) or lacosamide (Vimpat®), both anticonvulsants and mood stabilizers, can be used as an alternative to oxcarbazepine (Trileptal®) for youth who may not tolerate oxcarbazepine well. Less commonly used anticonvulsants are carbamazepine (Tegretol®) and levetiracetam (Keppra®), whereas divalproex sodium (Depakote®) is not recommended as it does not work as effectively as the others. For those taking lamotrigine (Lamictal®) or lacosamide (Vimpat®), 25–50 mg increases every 7–10 days is recommended. The weight-based dosing range for lamotrigine (Lamictal®) is 6–10 mg/kg/day with a recommended blood serum level of 10–12. The weight-based dosing range for lacosamide (Vimpat®) is 8–12 mg/kg/day with a recommended blood serum level of 10–15.

It's also important to note that puberty can change blood levels—the release of hormones can interfere with medication—so it may be necessary to check levels more frequently during this time. For example, estrogen released during menstruation is a convulsant and can work against the effects of an anticonvulsant. Puberty is a tough stage for anyone, but especially for kids with DMDD! Extra monitoring is needed and slight shifts in dosage may be frequent. During puberty, some children may also require medication to address anxiety and/or depression in addition to the Matthews Protocol.

Finally, it's worth nothing that while the medications used in the Matthews Protocol are FDA-approved, their application in treating DMDD is considered off-label. However, an increasing body of research and clinical experience supports the effectiveness of these medications in managing the symptoms of DMDD. The off-label use of these drugs in the Matthews Protocol is justified by their ability to stabilize mood, reduce irritability, and improve overall functioning in affected children.

Please note: the information provided here is for guidance only and should not be considered medical advice. The authors are not licensed prescribers. It is essential to consult and work closely with an experienced physician or nurse practitioner when considering or attempting any medications. Always seek professional medical guidance before making decisions about your health.

> For our daughter, the Matthews Protocol didn't work right away. It took approximately six months before my daughter reached a therapeutic range of oxcarbazepine. We were encouraged by other DMDD parents not to give up hope and to have patience, as it typically takes anywhere from three to six months to reach therapeutic levels. The longer she was on the therapeutic doses of the protocol, the less frequent her outbursts were becoming. She needed to get used to the way her brain was now functioning and there was an adjustment period for her and for us. Even though she was eight, she seemed to have an emotional skill level of a four-year-old because she did not learn those age-appropriate skills at a younger age when she dysregulated. Within the first year of being stable on the protocol, she had fully caught up and had emotional control similar to that of her peers. Timing of the protocol medication is particularly important, especially before blood labs. Oxcarbazepine or lamotrigine should be taken 12 hours apart and we had the best success when we followed this schedule as indicated. Obtaining regularly scheduled morning blood draws (12 hours after nighttime dose) for serum levels as our daughter grew helped us make small dosage adjustments to keep her stable in the suggested range. The first couple of years on the protocol, our daughter was part of the 25% of patients who benefit from a 48-hour amantadine break (done over a weekend when we would be home) every four to six weeks as needed to combat receptor exhaustion. Going off amantadine for a full 48 hours allowed the receptors to reset, and the medication would continue to work well again. These breaks were usually difficult but very much needed. For more detailed information about the protocol, visit the Revolutionize DMDD website, www.rdmdd.org, which has information not only for parents but also for medical providers, too.

Cognitive-Behavioral Therapy (CBT)

Cognitive-behavioral therapy (CBT) is a widely used therapeutic approach that has shown effectiveness in treating mood disorders, including DMDD. CBT focuses on helping the child identify and change negative thought patterns and behaviors that contribute to emotional dysregulation. Through CBT, children with DMDD can learn coping strategies for managing their anger and frustration, improving their emotional regulation, and reducing the frequency and intensity of their temper outbursts. CBT can also help children develop problem-solving skills and enhance their ability to navigate challenging situations without resorting to extreme emotional reactions.

Parent Training and Family Therapy

Given the significant role of environmental factors and particularly family dynamics in the development and maintenance of DMDD, involving parents and caregivers in the treatment process is essential. Parent training programs can equip parents with invaluable skills to better manage their child's behavior, implement consistent discipline strategies, and create a supportive home environment. Techniques such as positive reinforcement, clear communication, and setting consistent boundaries can help reduce the child's irritability and improve family relationships. Family therapy may also be beneficial in addressing any underlying family conflicts or issues that are contributing to the child's emotional dysregulation. By improving family dynamics, family therapy can create a more stable and supportive environment for the child, which in turn can help mitigate the symptoms of DMDD. Sam has developed an 11-session group program for parents that covers many of the topics introduced in this book.

School-Based Interventions

Since DMDD symptoms often manifest in school settings, school-based interventions are a crucial component of the treatment plan. Schools can provide structured environments that support the child's emotional and behavioral regulation. Interventions for eligible children are offered through individualized education plans (IEPs), including behavioral support programs and social skills training; these programs can help children with DMDD cope with the challenges of the school environment. Additionally, training teachers and school staff to recognize and respond appropriately to DMDD symptoms can prevent the escalation of outbursts and reduce the disorder's impact on the child's academic performance and their social relationships.

Early Intervention

Early intervention is vital in preventing the long-term adverse effects of DMDD—identifying and addressing the disorder in its early stages can prevent symptoms from becoming more severe and ingrained. Early intervention programs focusing on building emotional regulation skills, improving family dynamics, and supporting the child and their caregivers can significantly improve outcomes. These programs may include parent training, individual therapy for the child, and school-based interventions to address the disorder from multiple angles.

A Holistic Approach

A holistic approach to treatment that integrates pharmacotherapy, psychotherapy, family support, and school-based interventions will likely be most effective in managing DMDD. This approach recognizes that DMDD is a complex disorder with multiple contributing factors and that addressing these factors in isolation is unlikely to lead to sustained improvement. In contrast, by addressing the genetic, neurobiological, *and* environmental influences on DMDD, a holistic treatment plan can provide comprehensive support for the child and their family, leading to better long-term outcomes.

The Bottom Line

Raising a child with DMDD presents unique challenges that often feel overwhelming for parents. The unpredictable nature of severe temper outbursts and chronic irritability requires not only a deep understanding of the disorder but also a compassionate, patient approach to daily life. As this chapter has outlined, DMDD is not a condition that children can easily "outgrow" or one that will resolve without significant intervention. Instead, it's a complex disorder requiring a comprehensive, multifaceted approach to care. For parents, this means becoming both an advocate for their child's needs and a source of unwavering support.

Because DMDD is a relatively new diagnosis as of 2013—it's only been officially recognized in recent years—there's limited long-term data on the adult outcomes for children diagnosed with DMDD. While researchers continue to actively study the disorder, the trajectory from childhood to adulthood of people with DMDD remains unclear. Consequently, predictions about the long-term impacts of DMDD on behavior, mental health, and overall functioning are still being developed. As more studies are conducted, a clearer understanding of adult outcomes will emerge, helping to better inform treatments and support strategies for those affected by DMDD.

But one thing is certain: understanding DMDD is the first critical step for parents. When parents familiarize themselves with the symptoms, diagnostic criteria, and underlying causes of the disorder, they can more accurately recognize the signs of it and can seek early intervention, which is crucial for improving outcomes. Knowledge empowers parents to navigate the healthcare system effectively and ensure that their child receives appropriate assessments and treatments. Understanding DMDD also helps parents and clinicians distinguish between behaviors that result from the disorder and behaviors that are typical of other developmental stages and disorders, allowing for more tailored and effective responses.

An essential aspect for parents is adopting strategies that help manage their child's emotional and behavioral challenges. This often involves creating a structured and predictable environment at home, which can help reduce the frequency and intensity of outbursts. Consistent routines, clear expectations, and calm, consistent responses to behavior can significantly affect how a child with DMDD navigates their day.

Support systems are also vital. Parents should not hesitate to seek help through therapy, support groups, and/or educational resources. Connecting with other parents facing similar challenges can provide emotional support, practical advice, and a sense of community. Furthermore, involving the child's school in their treatment plan can ensure that they receive the necessary accommodations and support in the educational environment, which is often where symptoms of DMDD are most pronounced.

Of equal importance, parents need to practice self-care. Raising a child with DMDD can be exhausting and emotionally draining, and it's easy for parents to neglect their own needs. But despite this, maintaining their own mental and physical health is crucial for parents' well-being and their ability to care for their children effectively. Seeking counseling or therapy, engaging in stress-reducing activities, and ensuring they have time for themselves can help parents stay resilient and avoid burnout.

Finally, parents need to foster a hopeful and positive outlook. While DMDD does present significant challenges, with the proper support and interventions, many children with this disorder can go on to lead successful, fulfilling lives. By focusing on their child's strengths, celebrating small victories, and remaining patient and persistent in the face of setbacks, parents can help their child develop the skills they need to manage their emotions, build healthy relationships, and thrive despite the challenges of DMDD.

Final Words

Understanding DMDD is just the beginning for parents. The journey also involves learning about the disorder and actively engaging in strategies to support their child, seeking help when needed, and maintaining their well-being. With early intervention, comprehensive treatment strategies, and ongoing support, parents can significantly impact their child's ability to manage DMDD and improve their overall quality of life, creating a more harmonious and hopeful future for the entire family.

Raising a child with DMDD presents unique challenges—it requires parents to understand the disorder while fully embracing compassionate and structured strategies to address it. The upcoming chapters will provide parents with practical strategies for fostering emotional resilience, self-discipline, empathy, and effective communication while also offering tools to help their children navigate challenges, develop a growth mindset, and build on their strengths. These insights will empower parents to create a supportive environment that promotes their child's emotional stability and well-being as well as their own.

Chapter 3
The Eight Guideposts for Raising Emotionally Resilient Children with DMDD

Jonas' Story

Jonas Smith is a 13-year-old boy whose journey with DMDD has deeply affected his family. His mother Claire shared that Jonas should have been a healthy, happy child—her pregnancy was full-term and uncomplicated, and Jonas was raised in a stable home with two loving parents. Despite this, Jonas exhibited signs of frustration at an early age. Claire spent much of Jonas' first year telling herself, "He'll be happier when he can sit up, crawl, etc." Yet he never was. Just a few months after his first birthday, the rage began to flare up. Jonas would get angry often and he would want to hurt his mother—he would pinch her, pull her hair, and bite her.

By the time Jonas was a toddler, his chronic irritability and rage had become the norm in the family's life. His first sentence was "Throw shoes, Mama's face!" By the age of two, Jonas was adding verbal attacks to his physical ones, experiencing daily rages that could last nearly an hour. Despite these challenges, when Jonas wasn't raging, he and his mother had a close relationship: he liked to snuggle, he helped with chores, and he enjoyed reading books with her.

As Jonas approached preschool age, his rages continued; they seemed to lessen only temporarily. By his fourth birthday, the rages returned with full force, coinciding with his mother's pregnancy with his younger sibling. Jonas even started defecating and urinating in his bedroom during timeouts, adding to the chaos his family was enduring. Despite his outward appearance of being a model child—that was how his preschool teachers and other church members perceived him—Jonas's family saw a very different side at home.

When Jonas was eight, his family noticed that his behavior becoming more significant and involving physical threats to everyone. They sought a complete psychological evaluation, which led to a diagnosis of DMDD. Claire felt that the only reason Jonas qualified for the diagnosis was because he was homeschooled and home and school were essentially the same setting for him. His problematic behaviors weren't seen in settings outside of the home. Claire wondered—if Jonas were in a traditional school setting, would he display the same negative behaviors there that she was witnessing at home? If he didn't, would the diagnosis of DMDD have even been made? Claire couldn't help but consider this hypothetical scenario and if her son's problem behaviors were a result of poor parenting. This question haunted her.

> Once I learned what was happening in my son's brain that was causing his irritability and rages, I quickly found myself looking at his disorder from a different perspective. He wasn't acting out on purpose. He had an invisible illness and needed compassion, empathy, and a great deal of patience to help him through it. Having this knowledge, I was better able to educate family members, close friends, and teachers, who previously saw my son as having a behavioral issue instead of a neurological one.

As Jonas' story makes clear, raising a child with DMDD demands more than typical parenting skills—it requires a deep well of empathy, a consistent approach, and a nuanced understanding of the child's unique challenges. To that end, this chapter introduces eight essential guideposts designed to help parents foster emotional resilience in their children with DMDD. Each guidepost addresses different aspects of a child's development, offering practical strategies that parents can use to create a supportive home environment, manage symptoms effectively, and ultimately guide a child toward emotional stability and resilience.

Teaching and Conveying Empathy

Empathy is the cornerstone of emotional resilience, especially for children with DMDD. But empathy involves more than simply understanding a child's feelings—it requires making a deliberate effort to connect with them emotionally and acknowledging their experiences as being valid and significant. For Liam, a young boy whose emotions often escalated rapidly, learning empathy began with his parents modeling it daily in their interactions with him and others.

To better help their son, Michael and Sarah consciously tried to listen to Liam's frustrations without immediate correction or judgment. For instance, when Liam struggled with his math homework and became frustrated to the point of tears, they resisted the urge to fix the problem for him or dismiss his feelings. Instead, they sat beside him, acknowledged his frustration, and expressed an understanding of his struggle. This simple act of empathy helped Liam feel understood, reducing the intensity of his emotional outbursts.

Teaching empathy to a child with DMDD goes beyond addressing immediate emotional needs—it involves creating opportunities for the child to practice compassion toward others. Parents can encourage their children to engage in simple acts of kindness, such as helping a neighbor carry their groceries or caring for a pet. These activities allow children to experience the satisfaction of helping others, which reinforces their sense of connection to the world around them. For Liam, participating in a local community garden project where he could help plant flowers and vegetables became a regular activity. It provided a peaceful environment where he could engage with nature, and it also gave him a tangible way to contribute to something larger than himself.

Modeling empathic behavior in everyday situations also plays a critical role in teaching children with DMDD how to relate to others. When Michael and Sarah faced their challenges— whether it was a difficult day at work or dealing with a family issue—they discussed their feelings openly in front of Liam, demonstrating that everyone experiences emotions and that it's okay to express them. This transparency helped Liam understand that emotions are a normal part of life and that empathy is about supporting each other through these experiences.

Creating a home environment where empathy is regularly practiced and valued can significantly impact any child's emotional development, but it especially helps children with DMDD learn to manage their own emotions more effectively (while also understanding and relating to the feelings of others). As Liam grew older, the empathy he learned at home began to trickle into his interactions at school and with friends, making him more patient and less prone to outbursts when things didn't go his way.

Effective Communication and Listening Actively

Effective communication is the bedrock of any secure relationship, and it's especially crucial when parents are raising a child with DMDD. Raj and Priya initially struggled with their daughter's intense emotional reactions, but they found that active listening—truly hearing Anika's concerns without interrupting or jumping to solutions—created a safer space for her to express her feelings. This approach was transformative in their relationship, helping to ease tensions and reduce the frequency of Anika's outbursts.

But a caveat: active listening involves more than just hearing words—it requires engaging with a child on multiple levels. Raj and Priya learned to maintain eye contact with Anika when she was speaking, which helped convey that they were fully present and focused on her. They also used affirmative gestures such as nodding or softly saying "I understand" to encourage Anika to continue sharing her thoughts and feelings. Though seemingly minor, these small actions helped Anika feel valued and understood, a mindset that made her more willing to openly communicate.

One of the critical elements of effective communication is validating a child's emotions. When Anika expressed anger or frustration, her parents resisted the urge to offer solutions or correct her behavior immediately. Instead, they focused on validating her emotions by acknowledging them as being real and significant. For example, when Anika was upset after having had a conflict with a friend, Raj and

Priya would say, "It sounds like you're hurt by what happened. That could be really tough." This validation helped Anika feel supported, which often diffused her anger and opened the door for a more productive conversation.

Raj and Priya also improved their communication styles to support Anika better. They realized that their tone of voice, choice of words, and even body language significantly affected how their daughter responded to them. By adopting a calm, steady tone and avoiding accusatory language, they were able to de-escalate potentially volatile situations. For instance, instead of saying, "Why are you always so angry?", they learned to ask, "What happened that upset you today?" This shift in approach helped Anika feel less attacked and more understood, making her more receptive to their guidance.

> As a childhood cancer survivor, I distinctly remember the day of my diagnosis. I was brought to the doctor, tests were run, we were ushered to a small room, and our lives were swept off the ground. Resources, treatment plans, and respite/palliative care were all at our fingertips. Mental illness is different. Instead of having a path to follow, we were questioned and told our daughter would grow out of it. Instead of getting a list of resources, we had to find them ourselves. Instead of a firm treatment protocol, we spent years trying different medications that never really worked until we learned about the Matthews Protocol. Children with DMDD are missing out with the slow pace of diagnosis and treatment.

Effective communication also involves teaching a child how to express their feelings constructively, so Raj and Priya encouraged Anika to use "I" statements, such as "I feel upset when…" rather than "You always make me mad when…" This subtle shift empowered Anika to take ownership of her emotions and communicate them without immediately blaming others. Over time, Anika became more successful at expressing her feelings calmly and clearly, which helped reduce misunderstandings and conflicts at home and school.

Incorporating these communication strategies into daily interactions can significantly improve relationships between parents and children with DMDD. Parents can help their children develop the communication skills necessary for healthy emotional expression and stronger interpersonal relationships by creating a safe, open environment where feelings are respected and understood.

Accepting Children for Who They Are: Conveying Unconditional Love and Setting Realistic Expectations

Knowing that they are unconditionally loved and accepted is vital for children with DMDD, as they often struggle with self-esteem due to their intense emotional experiences. David and Elena, for example, faced the challenge of helping their daughter

Maya feel loved and accepted despite her frequent outbursts. They learned that expressing consistent affection and reassurance helped Maya feel secure and valued even after a brutal episode.

Children with DMDD frequently encounter situations where their emotions are overwhelming, leading to behaviors they don't fully understand. The unconditional love and acceptance of their parents become a crucial anchor in these moments. For David and Elena, this meant making certain that Maya knew she was loved no matter what. After an outburst, instead of focusing on her behavior, they focused on the emotional aftermath, offering comfort and reassurance. They often told Maya, "We love you and we're here for you no matter how tough things get." This unconditional support helped Maya recover more quickly from her emotional episodes and reduced her anxiety about disappointing her parents.

Setting realistic expectations is another essential aspect of fostering resilience in children with DMDD. David and Elena understood that holding Maya to the same standards as other children her age could lead to unnecessary stress and feelings of inadequacy, so instead, they adjusted their expectations to align with Maya's unique abilities and challenges: they set small, achievable goals that allowed her to experience success and gradually build her confidence. For instance, instead of expecting her to complete all of her homework in one sitting, they broke it down into smaller tasks with breaks in between. This approach helped Maya feel more capable and less overwhelmed, reducing her frustration and improving her ability to cope with challenges.

Celebrating small victories is another powerful way to reinforce a child's self-esteem. David and Elena made a point to acknowledge and praise Maya's efforts no matter how minor they seemed. Whether she stayed calm during a frustrating situation or she completed a small task without assistance, such moments were highlighted and celebrated. Focusing on what Maya did well rather than what she struggled with helped her build a positive self-image. Over time, this positive reinforcement contributed to Maya's resilience, giving her the inner strength to face her challenges more confidently.

Moreover, David and Elena were diligent in their attempts to understand the underlying reasons for Maya's behavior. They learned that her outbursts were often not just about the immediate trigger but were connected to deeper feelings of fear, insecurity, or frustration. They were then able to provide more effective support by addressing these root causes with empathy and understanding rather than reacting solely to the behavior she exhibited. For example, when Maya had a meltdown over a minor change in her routine, they realized that her fear of unpredictability was causing her distress. Maya gradually became more adaptable as her parents helped her understand that changes often occur and that they would support her through them.

By consistently conveying unconditional love and setting realistic expectations, parents can help their children with DMDD develop a strong sense of self-worth and resilience. This approach supports the child's emotional development. It also fosters a trusting, secure relationship between parent and child, which is essential for navigating the complexities of DMDD.

Nurturing "Islands of Competence"

Every child possesses strengths, or "islands of competence," that can be nurtured to build confidence and resilience. These strengths are often the key to helping children with DMDD develop a positive self-image, providing areas where they can excel and find joy. For Liam, his love for drawing became a crucial outlet. Michael and Sarah noticed that when their son was engaged in drawing, he was calmer and more focused, so they began to encourage this interest, providing him with art supplies and enrolling him in a local art class.

But nurturing these islands of competence involves more than just recognizing a child's strengths—parents need to create an environment where their child's strengths can flourish. Michael and Sarah made a concerted effort to integrate drawing into Liam's daily routine, ensuring that he had regular opportunities to engage in this activity. They also sought ways to expand his interest by exposing him to different styles and techniques, taking him to art museums, and introducing him to other artists. This nurtured his talent and helped him develop a sense of identity as an artist, which became a source of pride and confidence for him.

Focusing on these strengths allowed Liam to develop a positive self-image. He began to see himself not just as a child who struggled with intense emotions but as an artist with a unique talent. This shift in perception was crucial in building his resilience. Whenever he faced difficulties, whether in school or during social situations, he had something positive to anchor himself to—a talent that defined him beyond his challenges with DMDD.

Parents can further nurture their children's islands of competence by helping them set and achieve goals related to their strengths. For instance, Michael and Sarah encouraged Liam to enter local artwork competitions and share his creations with family and friends. These experiences validated Liam's abilities and gave him a sense of accomplishment and recognition from others. Each success, no matter how small, contributed to his growing self-esteem and belief in his ability to succeed despite his challenges.

In addition to nurturing existing strengths, parents can help their children discover new areas of competence. This involves exposing the child to various activities and interests, allowing them to explore different fields until they find something that resonates with them. For Liam, discovering his love of art was a turning point. Still, Michael and Sarah encouraged him to try new things like music and sports to see if any other interests might emerge. This approach broadens a child's horizons and increases their chances of finding other strengths that can be nurtured.

Nurturing islands of competence also involves teaching children to take pride in their accomplishments without becoming overly dependent on external validation, which is why Michael and Sarah emphasized the importance of self-satisfaction in Liam's achievements—they encouraged him to take pride in his work regardless of whether it won a prize or received praise from others. This internal sense of accomplishment helped Liam develop more resilient selfesteem, making him less vulnerable to the ups and downs of external feedback.

Parents can help children develop a more positive self-image, build resilience, and find joy in their abilities by focusing on and nurturing their strengths. This approach enhances children's emotional well-being and provides them with the tools they need to navigate the challenges of DMDD with greater confidence and stability.

Helping Children Learn from Rather Than Feel Defeated by Mistakes

Teaching children with DMDD to perceive mistakes as learning opportunities is crucial for bolstering their resilience. Mistakes are an inevitable part of life, but for children with DMDD, they can be particularly challenging. Anika, for example, often felt overwhelmed by her mistakes, which led to heightened anxiety and further outbursts. Raj and Priya realized that they needed to adopt a growth mindset approach that would emphasize effort over perfection and teach Anika that mistakes are a natural part of learning.

The first step in this approach was to change how they reacted to mistakes. Instead of focusing on what went wrong, they shifted their attention to what could be learned from the experience. When Anika made a mistake on a school project and became frustrated, Raj and Priya guided her through a reflective process, asking questions like "What part of this project do you think was most challenging?" and "What might you do differently next time?" This process helped Anika analyze her actions, identify areas for improvement, and develop a plan for handling similar situations in the future.

Raj and Priya also worked to model this growth mindset in their own lives—they shared stories with Anika about times when they had made mistakes and what they had learned from them. Showing her that everyone makes mistakes and that mistakes can lead to growth helped Anika feel less isolated in her experiences. For instance, Priya shared a story about when she had made an error at work but used the opportunity to improve her skills. This transparency helped Anika understand that making mistakes is not a sign of failure but rather a stepping stone to success.

To reinforce this mindset, Raj and Priya introduced a "mistake of the week" ritual at home, where each family member—including Anika—would share a mistake they had made and then tell everyone what they had learned. This practice normalized making mistakes and turned them into learning opportunities. It also helped Anika see that mistakes are not something to fear or be ashamed of—instead, they're an essential part of personal growth.

Additionally, Raj and Priya emphasized the importance of effort over innate ability, praising Anika for her hard work and persistence rather than just the outcome of her efforts. When Anika completed a challenging task, they said, "We're so proud of how hard you worked on this!" rather than focusing solely on the final result. This shift in focus helped Anika develop a sense of pride in her efforts, reducing her fear of failure and encouraging her to keep trying even when things didn't go perfectly.

This approach also extended to how Raj and Priya handled Anika's emotional outbursts. Instead of viewing these episodes as failures, they helped Anika reflect on what had triggered the outburst and what she could do differently next time. Over time, Anika learned to anticipate situations that might lead to frustration and developed strategies to manage her emotions before they escalated. This self-awareness and proactive approach to handling mistakes contributed significantly to her emotional resilience.

In short, parents can foster a growth mindset that encourages perseverance, resilience, and emotional stability by helping children with DMDD learn from their mistakes rather than feel defeated by them. This approach helps children manage their emotions more effectively, and it also helps them feel more confident about overcoming challenges and achieving their goals.

Teaching Children to Solve Problems and Make Sound Decisions

Problem-solving and decision-making are essential skills that children with DMDD need in order to become more independent and confident. That's because children with DMDD often feel overwhelmed by choices and challenges, which can then trigger their outbursts. Maya usually found herself paralyzed by indecision, something that only heightened her anxiety and frustration. To address this, David and Elena introduced a structured approach to problem-solving, helping Maya break down challenges into manageable steps.

The first step in teaching problem-solving was helping Maya identify the problem—when faced with a challenge, she often felt overwhelmed, making it difficult to pinpoint the specific issue that needed to be addressed. David and Elena worked with her to articulate the problem clearly and break it into smaller, more manageable parts. For example, if Maya was upset about a disagreement with a friend, they would help her identify the specific issue—was it about feeling left out, or had she not understood something her friend had said? Gaining this kind of clarity made the problem seem less daunting and more solvable.

Next, David and Elena guided Maya through brainstorming potential solutions. They encouraged her to think creatively and to consider both conventional and unconventional approaches. They taught her that there are often multiple ways to solve a problem and that brainstorming is about generating ideas without immediately judging them. This approach helped Maya feel more in control of the situation, as she realized that she did indeed have options and wasn't stuck with just one solution.

After brainstorming, the next step was to evaluate the pros and cons of each potential solution. David and Elena introduced a simple method: a pros and cons list. Together with Maya, they would list the advantages and disadvantages of each option, helping her weigh the potential outcomes. This critical analysis encouraged thoughtful decision-making and minimized making impulsive choices, a tendency that's common in children with DMDD. For example, if Maya was deciding whether or not to invite a friend over, she and her parents would discuss the pros (having fun and spending time together) and the cons (the possibility of getting into an argument).

Once a decision was made, David and Elena stressed the importance of implementing and monitoring the effectiveness of the chosen solution. They taught Maya to observe the results of her actions and reflect on what had worked well and what could be improved. This reflective practice enhanced Maya's problem-solving skills and built her resilience by demonstrating that adjustments could always be made if the initial solution hadn't worked as expected. If a less than optimal outcome had occurred, they would revisit the problem-solving process, encouraging Maya to try a different approach and not feel discouraged.

David and Elena also incorporated decision-making into everyday activities to reinforce these skills—they involved Maya in decisions about family activities, meal planning, and even household chores, giving her opportunities to practice problem-solving in a low-stakes environment. These experiences promoted Maya's confidence in her decision-making abilities, making her less likely to feel overwhelmed by more significant challenges.

Teaching problem-solving and decision-making skills also involved helping Maya develop coping strategies for when things didn't go as planned. David and Elena taught her techniques for managing disappointment and frustration, such as deep breathing, taking a break, or talking through her feelings. These strategies helped Maya recover more quickly from setbacks and approach problems with a calmer, more rational mindset.

By consistently applying this kind of structured approach to problem-solving and decision-making, parents can help their children with DMDD develop the skills they need to navigate through challenges more effectively. This in turn fosters greater independence and confidence and empowers children to better manage their emotions and actions, leading to more positive outcomes in their daily lives.

Disciplining in Ways That Promote Self-Discipline and Self-Worth

Effective discipline for children with DMDD focuses on fostering self-discipline and self-worth rather than relying on punitive measures that result in increased anger and resentment. Traditional disciplinary approaches that emphasize punishment can be particularly counterproductive for children with DMDD, as they may exacerbate feelings of frustration and low self-esteem. For example, Liam often struggled with understanding the consequences of his actions, which led to repeated negative behaviors. Michael and Sarah realized that they needed to shift their disciplinary approach to help Liam develop greater self-regulation skills.

They began by shifting from punitive measures to positive reinforcement. Instead of focusing solely on correcting Liam's negative behaviors, they started actively recognizing and rewarding his positive behaviors. For instance, when Liam managed to stay calm during a situation that typically triggered an outburst, they praised him for his self-control. This positive reinforcement helped Liam understand what behaviors were expected of him and thus made him more likely to repeat those behaviors in the future.

Michael and Sarah also maintained clear and consistent rules, thereby providing Liam with security and structure. Children with DMDD often thrive in environments where expectations are predictable and consistent—that stability reduces anxiety and helps them feel more in control. To ensure that Liam understood the rules, Michael and Sarah would explain them in simple and clear terms and regularly remind him of them in a calm, nonconfrontational manner. One of the rules was that when Liam felt overwhelmed, he could take a "cool-down" break in his room. This strategy gave him the space to manage his emotions without feeling punished.

Understanding the underlying reasons for Liam's behavior was another critical aspect of their approach to discipline. Michael and Sarah realized that Liam's outbursts often were based on his feelings of being misunderstood or overwhelmed. By addressing these root causes with empathy, they were able to provide more effective support. If Liam became upset during homework time, for example, instead of immediately disciplining him for his behavior, they would ask him what was bothering him and work together to find a solution. Maybe that was taking a break or approaching the task differently.

Michael and Sarah also introduced a system of natural consequences to promote selfdiscipline: rather than imposing arbitrary punishments, they allowed Liam to experience the natural consequences of his actions within a safe and controlled environment. If Liam refused to put away his toys, the natural consequence might be that he wasn't able to find them later when he wanted to play. This approach taught Liam that his actions had consequences and encouraged him to think more carefully about his choices.

In addition to natural consequences, Michael and Sarah used logical consequences directly related to the behavior in question. If Liam drew on the walls, the logical result would be that he needed to help clean it up. This approach was practical because it was fair and directly connected to the behavior, making it easier for Liam to understand and accept the consequences. Involving him in making amends also helped him develop a sense of responsibility and accountability for his actions.

In addition to all of the above, Michael and Sarah focused on maintaining Liam's dignity and self-worth during disciplinary moments. Instead of using shaming or punitive language, they communicated with their son in a way that affirmed his worth while still addressing his behavior—instead of telling him, "You're being bad," they would say, "We need to work on better ways to handle frustration." This approach helped Liam understand that although certain behaviors were unacceptable, just because he exhibited those behaviors didn't mean he was bad. This distinction was crucial in preserving Liam's self-esteem and encouraging him to strive for better behavior.

Parents can help their children with DMDD develop a more positive self-concept and better self-regulation skills by disciplining them in ways that promote self-discipline and selfworth. This approach reduces the frequency of negative behaviors. It also creates a more supportive and respectful relationship between parents and children, which is essential for children's emotional and behavioral growth.

Developing Responsibility, Compassion, and a Social Conscience

Teaching responsibility, compassion, and a social conscience helps children with DMDD understand the impact of their actions on others and also makes it easier for them to gain a sense of empathy and social responsibility, values that are crucial for helping children develop into well-rounded, socially aware individuals. For Anika—who often struggled with self-focus due to her intense emotional experiences—learning to consider the feelings and needs of others was a transformative process.

Raj and Priya introduced Anika to community service projects to help her develop a sense of responsibility and compassion. They started with small, manageable tasks, such as helping at a local food bank or participating in a neighborhood cleanup. These activities allowed Anika to see the positive effects that her actions had on others and gave her a sense of purpose. By helping her understand that she could make a difference in her community, Raj and Priya were able to shift her focus away from her own struggles and toward the needs of others.

Her parents also helped Anika develop a social conscience by involving her in discussions about social issues. They encouraged her to ask questions and express her thoughts about the world around her, helping her gain a greater sense of curiosity about and concern for others. For example, when Anika learned about the importance of recycling at school, her parents expanded the conversation at home by discussing the broader impact of environmental responsibility. That conversation helped Anika see that her actions could contribute to the greater good no matter how small her own actions happened to be.

Raj and Priya also used role-playing scenarios to help Anika practice empathy and compassion in a safe environment. They would create situations where Anika had to consider how someone else might feel in a given circumstance and decide how she would respond. This practice assisted Anika in developing the ability to perceive things from another person's perspective, something that's often challenging for children with DMDD to do. Over time, Anika became more adept at recognizing and responding to the emotions of others, both in role-playing scenarios and real-life situations.

Another critical aspect of developing responsibility and compassion is teaching children to take accountability for their actions. To that end, Raj and Priya encouraged Anika to reflect on how her behavior was affecting others and to take steps to make amends when necessary. Whenever Anika had an outburst toward a friend, her parents discussed the impact Anika's behavior had on her friend in a nonjudgmental way, and they also talked about a possible next step of Anika apologizing to her friend. Once Raj and Priya adopted this strategy, they saw that it helped their daughter take responsibility for her behavior.

To strengthen Anika's social conscience, Raj and Priya also involved her in family discussions about giving back to the community. They allowed Anika to help decide which causes or organizations the family would support, whether by donating to a charity, volunteering their time, or participating in a fundraising event. This involvement gave Anika a sense of ownership and pride in her family's efforts to make a positive difference, reinforcing her own growing sense of social responsibility.

> When we realized that our daughter had serious struggles with emotional regulation, we tried to improve her overall health and wellbeing in any way that we could. One of the first things we did was detox her body using Epsom salt baths, lymphatic massage, air purifiers, and water filtration systems. We tried to buy hormone-free milk and meats and to ensure that we only bought organic foods, especially those listed on the Dirty Dozen Guide, which are known to contain high levels of chemicals. We saw a neuropathic doctor who provided herbal drops to further detox under his guidance. We wanted to remove any potential things in the environment that could be contributing to her emotional outbursts. We also started limiting her access to digital devices and discovered "digital detoxing," where we would immerse her in outdoor activities and walks in nature. We found this "forest-bathing" to be helpful, not just for her brain but also for her body. She seemed much more relaxed and balanced at the end of the day after spending time exercising outside in nature. It also provided important time away from digital screens that we always felt were a trigger for her outbursts.

Teaching children with DMDD to develop responsibility, compassion, and a social conscience is a gradual process that requires patience and consistency. Parents can help children build a solid moral foundation and a greater awareness of the world by providing them with opportunities to practice these values in everyday life. This contributes to a child's emotional development and fosters a sense of connectedness and purpose, both of which are crucial for their overall well-being.

Returning to Jonas

After his diagnosis, Jonas began a series of medication trials. Sertraline (Zoloft®) made him hyperactive and disrupted his sleep, while oxcarbazepine (Trileptal®) did not help. Aripiprazole (Abilify®) initially brought some relief and made Jonas feel happy, but the effects were short-lived—his behavior soon deteriorated and that led to more physical aggression, although the severity of the rages lessened somewhat. Eventually, his parents agreed to have Jonas try lamotrigine (Lamictal®), but transitioning from aripiprazole to lamotrigine was challenging (they were aware that such a reaction was common). However, at the end of this difficult period, Jonas began to show improvement—he had more control over his anger even though he still struggled with irritability and impulsivity.

After Jonas' mother discovered the Matthews Protocol through a Facebook support group, she decided to explore that option. Jonas was already taking a lamotrigine, an anti-seizure medication and mood stabilizer that was working as expected by decreasing his irritability and improving his mood. With the approval of Jonas' psychiatrist, they added amantadine to his treatment plan. The results were remarkable: once Jonas was taking both medications, his irritability decreased significantly, he was less impulsive, and he began to smile and enjoy life. He was slower to react and respond to negative or unexpected situations. He had more time to think before reacting, which allowed him to make better decisions and avoid a meltdown or violent outburst.

Though things were much better for Jonas, he was still facing challenges. However, at that point in his journey, the strategies his parents had learned to guide and support him finally began to reap genuine benefits for all of them.

Final Thoughts and a Cautionary Note

In the following chapters, we'll extensively explore each one of the eight guideposts we introduced in this chapter, in the process offering a broad range of strategies and ways of overcoming obstacles. We designed these guideposts with practicality in mind—we wanted to give parents realistic strategies for raising emotionally resilient children with DMDD. While this journey is filled with unique challenges, these guideposts will serve as a roadmap that will allow families to effectively navigate their challenges. As we discuss each guidepost, we'll address the obstacles that often detract from success and we'll provide parents with the tools they need to overcome those obstacles.

Given how intertwined these eight guideposts can be, strategies for one guidepost may apply somewhat or just as much to several other guideposts, especially since all of the guideposts have a common goal: reinforcing a resilient mindset for children with DMDD.

By consistently applying these eight guideposts, parents can create a nurturing environment that empowers their children to cope with the complexities of DMDD with confidence and a stable outlook. The guideposts aren't just theoretical concepts—they're practical strategies that can be integrated into daily life, offering concrete steps that parents can take to support their child's emotional development.

For example, teaching empathy involves more than simply understanding a child's feelings. It requires parents to model empathic behavior, create opportunities for the child to practice kindness, and foster an environment where emotions are openly discussed and validated. Similarly, effective communication and active listening are critical for building trust and reducing the intensity of emotional outbursts. Parents will learn how to engage with their children in ways that make them feel heard and understood, which can significantly reduce the frequency and severity of DMDD episodes.

The guideposts also emphasize the importance of accepting children for who they are, nurturing their strengths, and teaching them to learn from their mistakes. These strategies help build a child's self-esteem and resilience, enabling them to face challenges more confidently. Parents can help their children develop a positive self-image and a stronger sense of self-worth by setting realistic expectations and celebrating small victories.

The guideposts encourage parents to focus on developing their children's problem-solving skills, teaching them to make sound decisions, and disciplining them in ways that promote self-discipline and self-worth. These skills are essential for children with DMDD to gain greater independence and emotional stability, both of which are crucial for them to have.

Ultimately, this comprehensive approach supports the child's emotional development and transforms the entire family—as parents consistently apply these guideposts, they'll witness a significant change in their children's ability to manage their emotions and navigate the complexities of life. This transformation fosters a future filled with hope and resilience, where both the child and family can thrive despite the challenges posed by DMDD.

We have articulated and applied the eight guideposts in our clinical and consultation work and have witnessed how helpful the eight guideposts can be when it comes to raising emotionally resilient children with DMDD. That said, we're also aware that children with DMDD can display impulsive, angry, out-of-control behaviors quite suddenly. At such times, the top priority for a parent is to ensure safety for the child and others. Given how quickly an explosive situation can arise, we believe the following cautionary note is warranted before we describe each of the guideposts in detail.

When navigating the complexities of raising a child with DMDD, parents need to be prepared to maintain a delicate balance between thoughtfulness and immediacy. Parents often acquire strategies that emphasize a calm, patient approach to dealing with their child's emotional challenges, carefully cultivating these methods over time. These techniques focus on prevention, reflection, and measured responses. However, in moments of acute crisis, parents must be prepared to act decisively, appreciating that sometimes swift intervention is necessary before words or preplanned strategies can be effective. When urgent situations arise—such as when a child's safety is at risk or emotions are spiraling out of control—*immediate* attention is needed. If a child is engaging in harmful behavior or if an emotional outburst escalates to the point of danger, parents cannot afford to wait! They must act quickly.

Interestingly, moments that require instant intervention don't contradict the significance of always having calm, reflective strategies foremost in mind. What's most important is that a parent is flexible when it comes to initiating different strategies— after all, different situations demand different responses. The ability to act quickly ensures that the situation is immediately stabilized, reserving conversations and processing for *after* the imminent threat has passed. Once parents have acquired this flexibility, they feel more confident in their decision-making skills.

Another cautionary note involves the irritability that often lingers between outbursts— that can make day-to-day interactions feel like everyone is walking on eggshells. This constant state of heightened tension means that there may be an undercurrent of unease even during calm moments. This might prompt parents to carefully consider whether or not to address issues at that exact time—sometimes leaving certain topics untouched during peaceful periods can prevent unnecessary escalation. Preserving the calm becomes another crucial tool in the parent's repertoire; they recognize that not every challenge needs to be confronted immediately, especially when a much-needed-but-fragile peace could be easily shattered.

Adopting the flexible approach that we're advocating will take time, and there will be setbacks along the way. But hopefully those setbacks will help parents gain a clearer understanding of what a child with DMDD requires at particular times and during particular situations.

Chapter 4
Teaching and Conveying Empathy to Children with DMDD

Patrick's Story

Patrick Adams was adopted at two weeks old, becoming the first of three children whom his parents would go on to adopt. Early on, they noticed quirks in his behavior, but friends and family reassured them that everything was normal. Patrick's mother Allison said, "He wouldn't sleep unless tightly swaddled, even after he started rolling over, and he required an utterly pitchblack room to sleep—any light would leave him awake for hours."

As Patrick grew, his behaviors became more concerning. He developed an impressive vocabulary early on but had a strange obsession with grotesque things. He appeared manipulative—he threw tantrums that lasted for hours—and he didn't respond to traditional discipline. "When he was angry, he would insult my husband and me with phrases like 'Eat poop!'" Allison shared. "At church, he would scream incessantly in the nursery, and if I held another child, Patrick would bite, scratch, and hit me until I put the child down."

Patrick's problematic behaviors followed him into preschool. He attended three different schools, two of which asked him to leave due to his conduct. "He refused to follow the rules, did not engage in any work that frustrated him, and mocked and physically hurt other students," said Allison. "One church-affiliated preschool even suggested doing an exorcism after Patrick drew a picture of drops of blood falling from a knife." At another preschool, he spent most of his time at home after having acted up in class; the classroom assistant eventually quit out of frustration. Despite his charm, extensive vocabulary, and quick wit, Patrick did not respond to discipline in any form, either at home or at school.

By kindergarten, Patrick's struggles had not diminished. "We were advised by the public school system that Patrick would eventually adjust to the new routine. Still, within weeks, we were called to start a behavioral intervention plan," said Allison.

Patrick couldn't keep his hands off other students and would threaten to harm teachers when they asked him to do something. In first grade, Patrick hit a teacher during recess and tried to run away from school. While school personnel were empathic, they initially resisted providing special education support—they first required an official diagnosis. Patrick's psychologist hesitantly diagnosed him with DMDD.

Empathy is a cornerstone of emotional resilience and can be very challenging for parents who have a child with DMDD. Such children often experience intense emotions that can overwhelm them, leading to frequent outbursts and a heightened sense of frustration. These emotional storms aren't just occasional occurrences but are part of daily life for many children with DMDD, making it essential for parents to approach their children with deep understanding and compassion—without empathy, parents might respond to their child's behavior with anger or frustration, and that's likely to exacerbate the child's emotional difficulties as well as strain the parent-child relationship. In contrast, empathy allows parents to connect with their children on an emotional level, acknowledging the child's feelings and helping them navigate their overwhelming emotions in a supportive and constructive manner.

This chapter will explore the critical role that empathy plays in raising emotionally resilient children, particularly those with DMDD. Empathy involves more than just understanding a child's emotions—it requires parents to demonstrate that understanding through their words, actions, and responses. For children with DMDD, the need for empathic parenting is even more pronounced as their emotional experiences are often more intense and less predictable than those of their peers. Empathy helps these children feel validated and supported, reducing the sense of isolation or misunderstanding that so often accompanies their condition.

In this chapter, we'll delve into practical strategies that parents can use to model empathy and nurture it in their children. One of the key strategies we briefly introduced in the previous chapter was active listening, where parents focus entirely on what their child is saying, both verbally and nonverbally, without interrupting or judging. This practice helps children feel heard and teaches them how to listen to others, laying the groundwork for developing empathy. Additionally, reflecting feelings to the child—such as saying, "It seems like you're feeling very angry right now"—can help children identify and understand their emotions, which is a crucial step in learning how to manage them.

Other important activities for nurturing empathy are role-playing and storytelling. Both allow children to practice seeing things from another person's perspective in a safe and supportive environment. Encouraging children to consider how others might feel in different situations helps them develop the ability to empathize with others even when their own emotions are intense.

Parents need to model empathy in their own behavior, not only in their interactions with their children but also in how they treat others. Children learn significantly from observing their parents! Consistent demonstrations of empathy can help them internalize this vital skill.

Finally, this chapter will highlight the importance of patience and self-care for parents. Empathy can be difficult to maintain, especially when dealing with the frequent and intense emotional outbursts that characterize DMDD. By caring for their own emotional and physical well-being, parents will be better equipped to approach their child's needs with the empathy and understanding their child needs for their emotional growth and resilience.

Teaching and conveying empathy to children with DMDD is not only beneficial, it's essential for fostering emotional resilience. By actively listening, reflecting feelings, modeling empathy, and taking care of themselves, parents can help their children navigate the challenges of DMDD with greater emotional strength and understanding.

The Importance of Empathy in Raising Resilient Children

Empathy is defined as the ability to understand the feelings of another. It's more than just a social skill—it's a foundational aspect of emotional intelligence. For children with DMDD, experiencing how their parents express empathy can significantly impact how they perceive and manage their own emotions. When a parent consistently demonstrates empathy, that fosters a sense of security and validation in the child, which is critical for their emotional development.

Take, for instance, the Brown family. Eight-year-old Liam's explosive outbursts often left his parents feeling overwhelmed and helpless. Initially, Michael and Sarah's attempts to discipline Liam focused on controlling his behavior rather than understanding its roots. It wasn't until they began to see the world through Liam's eyes—recognizing his frustration and confusion and realizing that he simply could not control his behavior when he became so agitated—that they could approach him with the empathy needed to calm him down and guide him through his emotional storms. This shift in perspective wasn't just pivotal, it was transformative in helping Liam learn to regulate his emotions more effectively.

Similarly, Raj and Priya were at a crossroads when their usual communication methods failed to reach their daughter. But by empathizing with Anika's perspective—her feelings of isolation and the overwhelming nature of her emotions—they could begin rebuilding trust and providing the emotional support she needed to navigate her mood swings.

Modeling Empathy: A Parent's Role

Parents are the primary role models for their children, and how they express and respond to emotions sets the tone for how their children will do the same. It's not just a role but a responsibility that parents can and should take on! For children with DMDD, this modeling becomes even more critical.

Consider Maya, whose sudden fits of anger and irritability became a significant concern for her parents. Initially, their response was one of frustration, a reaction that only exacerbated Maya's emotional distress. However, when David and Elena began to model empathy by acknowledging Maya's feelings—validating her anger and frustration while gently guiding her toward more appropriate ways of expressing these emotions—they noticed a gradual improvement in her behavior. Maya began to feel understood and supported, which reduced the frequency and intensity of her outbursts.

Parents can model empathy by employing many of the following strategies:

Active Listening

Active listening involves more than just hearing a child's words—it requires fully engaging with their verbal and nonverbal communication. For a child with DMDD who may be struggling with intense emotions, active listening can be a powerful tool to help them feel understood and valued. Parents can start by eliminating distractions when their child is speaking to them. This requires putting away phones, turning off the TV, and making eye contact; all of those actions tell the child that they have their parents' full attention. Nonverbal cues such as nodding or leaning slightly forward can also indicate that a parent is engaged in what their child is saying.

Another critical aspect of active listening is avoiding interruptions. Parents should allow their child to finish their thoughts without interjecting, even if they think they know what their child will say. This demonstrates respect and encourages children to express themselves more fully. Once children have finished talking, parents can paraphrase what they've said to ensure that they understand correctly—they might say, "It sounds like you're feeling upset because of what happened at school today." This confirms that parents have heard their children correctly and helps clarify their emotions.

In addition, parents should ask open-ended questions that encourage their child to explore their feelings and thoughts more deeply. Instead of asking a yes-or-no question like "Did you have a bad day?", a parent might ask "What was the hardest part of your day today?" This invites a child to share more details and opens up more meaningful dialogue.

By using these techniques, active listening becomes a way for parents to build trust and strengthen their emotional connection with their child.

Reflecting Feelings

Reflecting a child's feelings is crucial in validating their emotions and helping them cope with the complexities of their inner world. This is especially true for children with DMDD— when a child feels heard and understood, that can significantly reduce the intensity of their emotional outbursts. But reflecting feelings involves more than just repeating what a child has said! It's about connecting with the underlying emotions driving their words.

Parents can start by observing both verbal cues and body language. If a child says something like "I hate school!" and is visibly upset, parents might respond with "It seems like you're frustrated with what's happening at school right now." This communicates that the parent recognizes their child's words and the emotions behind them. Maintaining a calm and empathic tone is essential—a parent's response should be comforting rather than punitive.

In some cases, children might not have the vocabulary to express their feelings accurately. That's when parents should help them build their emotional vocabulary. For instance, if a child seems withdrawn after a playdate, their parent might say, "I noticed you're a bit quiet after your playdate. Are you feeling sad about something that happened?" Offering this cue helps children identify and label their emotions. This skill is precious for children with DMDD, who often experience emotional dysregulation. If a child won't share information about their day or even screams "Leave me alone!", then parents should not pursue asking the same question. Instead, they might simply and calmly say, "Okay. I like to hear about your day. Maybe you can tell me more about it at another time."

Demonstrating Patience

Demonstrating patience with a child who has DMDD is perhaps one of the most challenging yet essential aspects of parenting. Because children with DMDD often experience intense emotions that can lead to disruptive behavior, it's easy for parents to become frustrated or overwhelmed. However, responding as patiently as possible conveys a powerful message that their child's feelings are important and worthy of understanding even when they're expressed in challenging ways.

One strategy for demonstrating patience is for a parent to practice mindful breathing before responding to their child's outburst. Taking a few deep breaths can help a parent stay calm and avoid reacting impulsively, and maintaining a calm approach is crucial when dealing with a child who may already be in a heightened emotional state. This pause can give a parent a moment to consider their response and choose one that's supportive rather than punitive. However, a caveat: as we emphasized previously, if a child is experiencing a meltdown and displaying behaviors that might prove dangerous to themselves or others, a parent's first priority must be to ensure everyone's safety rather than begin a discussion with the child about their behavior.

Another aspect of patience is recognizing that emotional regulation is a skill that takes time to develop, especially for children with DMDD. Rather than expecting immediate compliance or understanding, parents must approach each situation as a learning opportunity. For instance, if a child is having a meltdown because they didn't get their way, parents should attempt to lessen their own anger and frustration and say, "I understand this is hard for you. Let's take a moment to calm down together." This approach models patience and teaches a child how to manage their emotions over time.

Celebrating small victories and a child's progress with regulating their emotions is essential no matter how minor those victories may seem. Acknowledging such moments helps reinforce positive behavior and shows children that their parents notice and appreciate their efforts even when they're struggling. Over time, consistent patience can help a child feel more secure and supported, reducing the frequency and intensity of their emotional outbursts.

Finally, it's important to remember that demonstrating patience also involves having selfcompassion. Parenting a child with DMDD is incredibly demanding, and there will inevitably be moments when parental patience wears thin. When this occurs, parents should strive to forgive themselves and recognize that they're doing their best in a challenging situation. Also, parents should always keep in mind that they must take care of their own emotional health in order to maintain the patience they'll need to support their child.

Teaching Empathy to Children with DMDD

Teaching empathy to children with DMDD involves more than just explaining the concept of empathy or introducing a strategy for children to gain more of it—teaching empathy requires consistent practice and reinforcement in daily interactions. Here, we've included some strategies to help nurture empathy in a child. Note that these strategies will be most effective when parents use them during the quieter moments in a child's life. After all, it's difficult for children to learn when their ability to use their executive functioning is being overwhelmed by strong emotions.

Labeling Emotions

Labeling emotions is a foundational step in helping children to develop emotional intelligence, especially children with DMDD. Many of them struggle to understand and articulate their feelings, which leads to frustration and outbursts. Helping a child identify and name their emotions provides them with the tools they need to understand their internal experiences more clearly and express them more constructively. For instance, instead of simply reacting negatively to a child's tantrum, parents might say, "It looks like you're feeling very upset right now. Maybe when things calm down, we can figure out what to do so that you don't feel as upset." That kind of statement helps children connect their physical sensations with their emotional state and also validates their feelings, conveying to them that it's okay to feel upset.

To expand on this strategy, parents might consider using an emotion chart with faces depicting various emotions: from anger and sadness to joy and surprise. Ask a child to point to how they feel during different situations. This visual aid can make it easier for them to identify and label their emotions, especially in moments when it would be challenging to verbally express those feelings.

Parents can also model expressing their feelings by openly labeling their emotions throughout the day. For example, a parent might say, "I'm feeling frustrated because I lost my keys, but I'm going to take a deep breath and keep looking." This not only teaches a child that everyone has emotions, but it also demonstrates healthy ways to cope with them.

As children become more familiar with labeling their emotions, they should be encouraged to use this skill in various contexts. For example, after a playdate, parents can ask a child how they felt when playing with their friend or how they think their friend felt. This ongoing practice reinforces the connections between emotions and experiences, helping children develop a more nuanced understanding of their emotional world. Over time, they'll be better equipped to articulate their feelings rather than resort to disruptive behavior. That's a significant step forward for children with DMDD!

Role-Playing

Role-playing is a powerful tool for teaching empathy, especially for children with DMDD and any child who may struggle to understand the perspectives of others. By engaging in role-playing activities, children can practice putting themselves in someone else's shoes, an essential ability when it comes to developing empathy. Parents can create scenarios where their child plays the role of someone who's sad, scared, or frustrated, and then parents can ask their child to express how they think that person feels and what they could do to help. Or parents might role-play a situation where a friend feels left out during a game and can then ask their child how they think the friend feels and what they could do to include them.

To make role-playing more effective, parents can begin with simple, relatable scenarios that their child encounters daily. For example, parents can role-play a situation where they forgot to do their homework and they have to explain that to the teacher. Children can consider how they would feel in that situation and how they would like the teacher to respond. This gives them a chance to practice empathy within a context that feels relevant and real.

Role-playing can also be incorporated into a child's daily routine by using puppets, dolls, or action figures to act out different emotional scenarios. This can make the activity more engaging and less intimidating, especially for younger children. A parent can also switch roles, allowing their child to assume the role of the parent or teacher while the parent acts as the child. This reversal can offer children a deeper understanding of the ways in which their actions might affect others and how different perspectives can influence emotions.

Another good opportunity to use role-playing is to prepare children for challenging situations, such as visiting the dentist or dealing with a conflict at school. By practicing these scenarios in a safe, controlled environment, children can develop strategies for managing their emotions and responding empathically to others in real life. Role-playing helps children with DMDD develop empathy and become more confident about handling various social situations, thus reducing the likelihood of emotional outbursts.

Encouraging Perspective-Taking

Encouraging perspective-taking is a crucial part of teaching empathy to children, particularly those with DMDD. Perspective-taking involves helping a child understand that others may have different thoughts, feelings, and experiences. This insight allows children to see beyond their immediate reactions and consider the impacts of their actions on others. One effective strategy to enhance perspective-taking skills is for parents to ask open-ended questions during and after social interactions. For example, if a child argues with a sibling or friend, parents can ask, "How do you think your friend felt when you took the toy?" or "What do you think your sibling felt when you said that?"

These questions prompt children to reflect on the situation from another person's point of view, a skill that's especially important for children with DMDD, who may struggle with emotional regulation and empathy. Over time, this practice can help them pause and consider others' feelings before reacting, leading to more thoughtful and less impulsive behavior.

Another strategy is to use everyday situations as teaching moments for perspectivetaking. For instance, if a parent witnesses someone being kind or unkind in a TV show while watching the show with their child or if a character exhibits those tendencies in a book they're reading together, the parent can ask their child how they think the characters feel and why. This reinforces the idea that everyone has their own perspective and helps a child practice empathy in a low-pressure setting.

Parents can also model perspective-taking in their interactions with others. For example, if someone cuts in front of them in line at the supermarket, instead of reacting angrily, the parent might say to their child, "I wonder if that person is in a hurry because they have an emergency?" When parents verbalize their thought processes, they show their child how to consider different perspectives and respond empathically even in frustrating situations.

Encouraging perspective-taking can also involve collaborative problem-solving. When a child is upset with someone, parents can sit down with the child and brainstorm ways to resolve the conflict that take the emotions of both parties into account. This encourages a child to see things from another person's viewpoint and teaches them that understanding the perspectives of others can lead to more constructive and peaceful solutions.

Praising Empathic Behavior

Praising empathic behavior is a must for reinforcing empathy in children, especially those with DMDD. Positive reinforcement helps children appreciate the value of their actions and motivates them to continue practicing empathy. When a child shows a tiny act of kindness, parents should acknowledge this behavior immediately with specific praise! If a child shares their toys with a sibling or comforts a friend who's upset, a parent might say "I really appreciate how kind you were to share your toys with your brother!" or "It was very thoughtful of you to comfort your friends when they were sad."

Specific praise is more effective than general statements because it identifies the exact behavior that parents want to encourage. Instead of saying a more general "Good job!", it's better to clearly identify what positive thing the child did—that helps them understand why their actions were necessary. Over time, this allows a child to internalize specific behaviors and view them as part of their identity.

It's also essential to celebrate empathic behavior publicly within the family. For instance, during family meals or gatherings, a parent might highlight—with obvious pleasure!—a situation where their child displayed empathy. This reinforces the child's behavior and sets a positive example for siblings and other family members.

Finally, parents should model self-praise by acknowledging their own empathic actions in front of the child. Parents might say, "I felt good about helping our neighbor today! Seeing them smile after I helped them with their groceries was nice." This comment emphasizes empathy as being a valuable trait and shows children that it's okay to feel proud of themselves for being kind and considerate to others.

Storytelling and Books

Storytelling and books are powerful tools for teaching empathy to children, particularly those with DMDD, as those children may need extra help with understanding and processing emotions. Stories allow children to see the world through the eyes of different characters, and that can help them develop empathy by fostering an understanding of various perspectives and emotional experiences. When choosing books, parents should select stories that highlight characters who are dealing with different emotions, making decisions, and/or resolving conflicts in ways that emphasize understanding and kindness.

After reading a story, it's helpful to engage a child in discussing the characters' feelings and actions. Parents can ask open-ended questions such as "How do you think the character felt when that happened?" or "What would you have done if you were in their shoes?" These questions encourage a child to reflect on the emotions and perspectives of others, an activity that's crucial for developing empathy. Parents reading a story about a character who's being bullied can ask their child how they think that character felt and how they could help someone in a similar situation.

Relating a story's themes to real-life situations that their child might encounter can be very beneficial. If a character in a book helps a friend, a parent might ask, "Have you ever helped a sad friend? How did that make you feel?" These kinds of questions help children connect the story with their own experiences, reinforcing the lesson of empathy in a personal and relevant way.

In addition to traditional books, parents might consider using stories from various media sources, such as audiobooks, movies, or even video games with vital narrative elements. Varying the formats can keep the learning process fresh and exciting.

Parents can also encourage their children to create their own stories through writing or drawing. Children can create characters and scenarios where empathy plays a central role, such as a character who helps others or resolves conflicts peacefully. This exercise not only reinforces the concept of empathy but also allows children to express their understanding in a way that's meaningful to them.

Finally, making storytelling a regular part of a child's routine can be very helpful. Parents might set aside time each day or week to read and discuss stories together. This consistent practice strengthens a child's understanding of empathy, plus it fosters a love of reading and deeper connections between parents and children. Through stories, children can learn that empathy isn't just a conceptual lesson to be learned but a way of understanding and interacting with the world around them.

The Struggle for Parents to Remain Empathic

Despite their best intentions, parents may find it challenging to remain empathic in the face of their child's intense emotional outbursts. Several obstacles can hinder empathy, including stress, fatigue, and the natural human tendency to react defensively when confronted with challenging behavior. For instance, Sarah struggled to stay empathic during Liam's outbursts, especially when she was tired from a long day at work. It wasn't until she recognized her limitations and took steps to manage her stress—such as practicing self-care and seeking support from her spouse—that she could approach Liam's emotional needs with the empathy he required.

Similarly, Priya lost patience with Anika's frequent mood swings. However, she found that by focusing on her own emotional well-being and taking breaks when needed, she could maintain her empathy and respond more effectively to Anika's needs. The following are obstacles to empathy that parents frequently face as well as several strategies to manage them effectively:

Feeling Stressed and Overwhelmed

Feeling stressed and overwhelmed are the most significant challenges to being an empathic parent. When parents are under constant pressure—whether due to work, financial concerns, or the demands of daily life—it becomes increasingly difficult to remain patient and empathic, particularly when confronted with a child's intense emotional outbursts. A parent who has just completed a stressful day at work may find it difficult to shift gears and respond calmly when their child has a meltdown. In such situations, the parent's stress levels can exacerbate the child's distress, creating a negative feedback loop where both parties feed off each other's emotions.

Parents need to develop strategies to decompress and recharge in order to manage their stress and remain empathic. This might include taking short breaks, practicing mindfulness, or engaging in relaxing activities such as yoga, meditation, reading, or listening to music. Sarah realized she was more prone to losing her temper with Liam after a tough day, so by incorporating a few minutes of deep breathing exercises before engaging with her son after work, she was better equipped to handle his emotional needs with patience and understanding as opposed to acting impulsively.

> One of the hardest things I learned as a DMDD parent was learning to slow down and focus on my mental well-being. I enjoy staying busy with many different things, but doing so left me over-extended and stressed most of the time. I was not in the right mindset to handle my son's outbursts. When a large toy car was thrown at my head, I wanted to hurl it back at him. Then, I realized I needed to reduce my responsibilities and focus on my state of mind. I needed to be the best version of myself for my child to be able to be the best version of himself.

Fatigue

Fatigue is another common barrier to empathy, particularly for parents of children with DMDD who may experience frequent disruptions to their sleep or encounter ongoing demands that are mentally and physically exhausting. Not surprisingly, when a parent is tired, their capacity to respond with empathy diminishes because they're operating with reduced emotional and cognitive resources. After a night of broken sleep due to a child's nightmares, a parent might find it challenging to muster the patience needed to address a tantrum the following day. This can produce a cycle in which fatigue reduces empathy. That in turn may exacerbate the child's behavior, leading to even more fatigue.

Parents can combat this negative cycle by prioritizing rest and sleep whenever possible and seeking support when they feel overwhelmed. For example, Priya noticed that after a particularly exhausting day, she was far more likely to lose her patience when Anika experienced mood swings. By ensuring that she got to bed earlier on those tiring days and occasionally asking her spouse to take over during particularly tough moments, Priya could maintain the empathy Anika needed despite being fatigued. This proactive approach not only helped Priya manage her exhaustion, it also provided her with a sense of relief and comfort because she knew that she wasn't alone in her struggles.

Defensive Reactions

Parents are naturally inclined to protect themselves. This defensive tendency can become an obstacle to empathy, particularly when they feel like their authority or parenting skills are being challenged by their child's behavior. When a child with

DMDD lashes out, it's easy for a parent to take the behavior personally, leading to feelings of anger or frustration. This defensiveness can manifest as impatience, harsh responses, or an attempt to assert control, all of which undermine empathic communication. For example, when Liam would scream or throw things during an outburst, Sarah sometimes felt like he was attacking her personally, and that triggered a defensive rather than empathic response.

To overcome this obstacle, parents should remind themselves that their child's behavior is a symptom of their emotional struggles, not a personal affront. Reframing the situation helps shift the focus from the parent's feelings to the child's needs. Sarah embraced this concept and worked on reminding herself that Liam's outbursts were not intentional attacks but rather expressions of his frustration and inability to cope. By depersonalizing these interactions, she was able to respond more calmly and empathically, even when Liam's behavior was provocative.

Inconsistent Boundaries

Another obstacle to empathy can occur when parents confuse being empathic with being overly permissive. The two are not the same! Empathy allows parents to place themselves in their child's shoes and become more effective in choosing a clear and consistent disciplinary practice that promotes self-discipline. Opting for an overly permissive approach would likely backfire, as a child with DMDD can become even more unsettled when parents adopt a style that lacks clarity and consistency. Children with DMDD benefit from structure and predictability. Still, Priya initially struggled with how much leniency to offer Anika during her mood swings— she worried that being too strict would exacerbate her daughter's distress.

The key is to establish and maintain boundaries that are both firm and compassionate. This involves communicating expectations clearly while also acknowledging the child's feelings. Priya found that empathy allowed her to be *more* effective, not less, in enforcing boundaries; she was able to calmly explain the rules and consistently apply them. She would also take the time to understand and validate Anika's emotional state, saying things like, "I understand that you're upset, but it's still important to follow the rules." This approach helped Anika feel secure and understood rather than controlled or dismissed.

Past Parenting Experiences and Guilt

Parents often bring their own childhood experiences and emotions into their parenting, enhancing or hindering their ability to empathize with their children. Parents who experienced a lack of empathy or harsh discipline during their formative years may struggle to be empathic with their own children, especially if they have unresolved issues themselves. Additionally, guilt—whether from past mistakes in parenting or from feeling inadequate—can cloud a parent's ability to be present and empathic in the moment. A parent who was frequently criticized as a child might react defensively to their own child's criticism and find it difficult to respond with understanding.

Addressing this obstacle requires self-reflection and sometimes professional support. Parents must acknowledge and work through their emotions and past experiences to avoid projecting them onto their children. When Priya felt guilty for not being more patient with Anika, for example, she began to reflect on what had prompted her own emotions and kept reminding herself that she was doing her best. In such situations, parents might find it very helpful to talk with a therapist or join a support group to understand and face these feelings.

Significant Disciplinary Differences Between Parents

It's not unusual for parents to have different disciplinary styles. As a result, they might respond in contrasting ways to their child's behavior. In many instances, these differences are relatively small and parents are able to come together to create a more consistent disciplinary approach, but these differences can become more pronounced when parenting a child with DMDD. One parent may accuse the other of being overly harsh and arbitrary; the other may then assert that they *have* to be increasingly harsh given how permissive their partner is being.

These different perspectives become even more hardened when parenting a child with DMDD whose moods and behaviors become more intense and unpredictable. When significant differences in disciplinary styles continue, parents should seek professional help to gain a better understanding of their child's behavior and to consider the most effective disciplinary techniques. The better parents understand how to raise and discipline a child with DMDD, the more likely the child's behavior is to improve.

> When my child becomes dysregulated, my entire body feels as though air is being sucked out of me without warning. Every fiber in my body stiffens while my heart beats intensely and rapidly. Simultaneously, my mind goes into overload thinking about what I need to do to stay calm, keep everyone safe, and help my son so the situation doesn't escalate. Unfortunately, my body and mind know this experience all too well. As I give my child space to calm his emotions, I retreat to a room in our house to get myself back to baseline. I often rely on deep breathing and EFT (Emotional Freedom Technique) tapping, which quickly lowers my cortisol and can be done anywhere.

Additional Strategies to Overcome Obstacles to Empathy

Self-Care

Self-care is essential for parents raising a child with DMDD, as it directly impacts their ability to manage the unique challenges associated with the disorder. Parents attending to their own emotional and physical health will be in a better position to support their child. As noted earlier, prioritizing sleep is crucial! A well-rested parent can think more clearly, respond more calmly to emotional outbursts, and maintain a positive outlook even during difficult times. Establishing a regular sleep routine, avoiding caffeine and screens before bed, and creating a relaxing bedtime environment can all improve sleep quality. Since sleep is essential for the brain, it's important for *everyone* in the family (but especially the child with DMDD) to have a regular sleep schedule.

Physical activity is another critical component of self-care. Regular exercise—whether a morning jog, a yoga session, or even a short walk—can reduce stress, boost mood, and increase energy levels. Incorporating exercise into one's daily routine benefits physical health and provides a valuable outlet for managing stress and anxiety.

Nutrition also plays a significant role in our overall well-being. A balanced diet with plenty of fruits, vegetables, whole grains, and lean proteins can help stabilize mood and energy levels. It's just as important to stay hydrated and avoid relying on excessive caffeine or sugary snacks—those can lead to energy crashes and irritability.

On top of those essentials, parents would be well-served by allocating time for activities that bring them joy and relaxation, such as reading, gardening, or pursuing their favorite hobbies. Engaging in these activities provides parents with an opportunity to recharge and maintain balance. Self-care is not selfish, it's necessary! It allows parents to be more effective caregivers for their children and be more able to meet the demands of parenting a child with DMDD with patience and empathy.

Seeking Support

Seeking support is a vital strategy for parents raising a child with DMDD. The challenges of managing frequent emotional outbursts and intense mood swings can be overwhelming! It's crucial to reach out to others for help. One of the first steps parents can take is to connect with friends and family who understand their situation and can offer emotional support. Even a simple conversation with a trusted friend can provide a sense of relief and help a parent feel less isolated. These conversations can also provide fresh perspectives on coping strategies, as others might share similar experiences or suggest new approaches to managing a child's behavior.

In addition to that kind of informal support, parents should consider joining a support group specifically for parents of children with mood disorders or behavioral challenges. These groups can be a valuable resource—they offer a community of individuals who truly understand the parent's unique difficulties. Sharing experiences in such a setting can be both cathartic and educational as parents exchange tips and resources and encourage others who are navigating similar journeys.

Professional support is also crucial—parents shouldn't hesitate to seek help from a therapist or counselor for themselves or as a family. A mental health professional can provide tailored advice and coping strategies, helping parents manage the stress and emotional toll that often accompanies parenting a child with DMDD. Family therapy can also improve communication and relationships within the household, thus creating a more supportive environment for the child with DMDD.

Lastly, parents benefit from making use of educational resources: books, webinars, and workshops on DMDD and related parenting strategies can provide valuable tools and knowledge. The more informed parents are about the disorder, the better equipped they'll be to advocate for their child and implement effective strategies at home. Seeking support in these various forms can significantly reduce the burden of parenting a child with DMDD, making the journey more manageable and less isolating.

Mindfulness Practices

Mindfulness practices can be a game changer for parents raising a child with DMDD— such techniques can help them remain calm, centered, and present even amid their child's emotional storms. Mindfulness involves paying deliberate attention to the present moment without judgment, which can be incredibly helpful when dealing with the unpredictable nature of DMDD.

One of the simplest and most effective mindfulness techniques is deep breathing. When a child is having an outburst, taking slow, deep breaths can help parents stay calm and prevent their own emotions from escalating. This practice calms the nervous system and models a healthy coping mechanism for children.

Meditation is another powerful mindfulness practice. Even 5–10 minutes of daily meditation can help develop greater emotional resilience and a clearer mind! Parents can begin their day with a short meditation, focusing on their breath or repeating a calming mantra. Over time, this practice can help parents approach challenging situations with more patience and less reactivity.

In addition to formal meditation, parents can incorporate mindfulness into everyday activities. They can practice mindful walking by focusing on the sensation of their feet touching the ground and the rhythm of their steps, for example. During meals, parents might engage in mindful eating by savoring each bite and noticing the flavors and textures. These simple practices can help ground parents in the present moment, making it less challenging to cope with the stresses of parenting a child with DMDD.

Taking short mental breaks throughout the day is also essential. When parents are feeling overwhelmed, it can be very therapeutic for them to step away for a moment, take a few deep breaths, and recenter themselves before reengaging with their child. These breaks can prevent burnout and help maintain the empathy and patience needed to support the child.

A Few Words About Siblings

Raising a child with DMDD presents unique challenges that affect the entire family, especially siblings. Parents must acknowledge and understand the emotional toll that DMDD can have on siblings and actively support their well-being and resilience, too, while simultaneously helping them have empathy toward their sibling with DMDD. The following strategies can help accomplish this task:

First, create a space where siblings feel safe to express their feelings. They may experience confusion, frustration, or resentment about their sibling's behaviors. Active listening—where parents validate emotions without judgment—helps siblings feel understood and valued. For example, saying, "It seems like you feel upset when your brother has a meltdown. It's okay to feel that way!" can open pathways for honest communication.

Educate siblings about DMDD in an age-appropriate way. Helping them understand that their sibling's outbursts result from their condition rather than them being deliberate actions fosters empathy. Use simple metaphors or storytelling to make complex emotional challenges relatable—for instance, comparing a sibling's emotional state to a storm that passes can help frame the situation as temporary and manageable. Or parents might say that the storm appears regularly but that people become better prepared for coping with storms. The story can also include the message that over time, the storm will become less intense and less frequent.

It's also key for siblings to receive quality one-on-one time with their parents—moments of undivided attention from their parents affirm their importance within the family and reduce feelings of neglect. Parents can engage in enjoyable and stress-free activities with siblings, thereby creating a more balanced household dynamic.

Parents can encourage siblings to engage in empathy-building activities like role-playing or shared storytelling. They can discuss how siblings might offer support during challenging moments or use their unique strengths to contribute positively to the family dynamic. Acts of kindness among siblings should be celebrated—that will reinforce collaborative and supportive relationships. When indicated and during calm moments, role-playing or shared storytelling should include the sibling with DMDD.

Finally, parents should seek professional support if siblings show stress or behavioral changes. Attending counseling or support groups tailored for families dealing with DMDD can offer siblings a broader understanding of their role and can give them strategies to cope with the emotional complexities of their family life.

By fostering open communication, empathy, and a supportive environment, parents can help siblings of children with DMDD thrive despite (or even because of) their family challenges.

A week before my daughter's allergy testing, she had to be off all antihistamines. She had been on Zyrtec for a year and when we stopped the medication, my husband and I noticed her mood was significantly better, even though her allergies were worse. When we were able to resume the antihistamine, we tried Xyzal. The next day, my daughter had a fight-or-flight situation, which she had not had in years. I decided to test her oxcarbazepine level the next day since I thought perhaps her level (she's been on Matthews Protocol) was low and contributed to her rage. To my surprise, her level was within therapeutic range and I concluded that the fight-or-flight was a direct result of the antihistamine. When I read that some adults had severe side effects that dramatically altered their mood while taking certain antihistamines, I realized this is more common than I thought. I since discovered that a Diamine Oxidase (DAO) enzyme effectively lowered her histamines, without negatively impacting her mood.

Back to Patrick

During the fall of Patrick's kindergarten year, the Adams adopted their third son. "We wanted our second son to have a companion," Allison explained. "But it wasn't safe to leave Patrick alone with the baby or the toddler—he wouldn't follow instructions and he intentionally subjected them to harm when I wasn't looking." Both Allison and her husband felt like it was a constant juggling act to keep everyone safe. "My toddler would sense one of Patrick's rages coming on and would carry the baby into his room to protect them both," she shared.

Now nine and six years old, the two younger boys both try to have a relationship with their older brother. "They're rightfully cautious and quick to find blame," Allison pointed out. "They've attended therapy to process traumatic events caused by Patrick's outbursts."

With an educational plan in place, the school implemented various strategies to help Patrick: smoother transitions between activities, breaks from the classroom, scheduled check-ins with a counselor, and enrollment in social skills classes. "Those measures helped for a while, but as soon as the novelty wore off, Patrick's old behaviors returned," said Allison. His parents fought to establish an Individualized Education Plan (IEP), a more formal agreement that provided specific goals and access to a paraprofessional aide who could help Patrick process things if needed. The school even paired Patrick with a child with autism to mentor. That facilitated Patrick's ability to gain more empathy—being a mentor allowed him to focus on someone other than himself. Patrick excelled academically, testing into the program for academically and intellectually gifted students. However, his behavioral issues persisted.

Patrick's parents turned to Facebook to search for help and answers. They discovered a support group and information about a promising protocol that Dr.

Matthews had developed for treating DMDD. At first, Patrick's psychiatrist was hesitant to try this unconventional treatment, but the psychiatrist eventually agreed. "After starting the first medication [oxcarbazepine], we noticed a slight improvement—his rages were reduced to two or three times a week instead of daily," Allison recalled. "When the doctor added the second medication [amantadine], Patrick's behavior improved dramatically within just three days! He became agreeable and calm and was rage-free for nearly two weeks."

Over time, Patrick's rages were reduced to only twice a month; each lasted 30–45 minutes and was less intense. School life improved, and Patrick began making friends and even getting invited to playdates. Despite an occasional setback, Patrick became what his parents called "stable." Although he still had struggles, they were nothing like the daily terrors they had all faced.

Final Words

Raising a child with DMDD is very challenging. However, interacting with their child gives parents an opportunity to foster deep emotional connections with their child and teach them valuable life skills. By consistently modeling and teaching empathy, parents can help children develop the emotional intelligence they need to cope with intense feelings and build stronger, more positive relationships with others.

Michael and Sarah found that Liam's outbursts became less frequent and more manageable as they became more attuned to Liam's emotional needs. With her parents' guidance, Anika learned to express her feelings more constructively, reducing the tension in her household. Maya benefited from her parents' empathic approach, which helped her regain some of the joy and stability she had previously lost to her volatile moods.

Their stories highlight the transformative power of empathy in managing the challenges posed by DMDD. By committing to showing empathy as a daily practice, parents can create a more harmonious home environment, support their child's emotional growth, and lay the foundation for a resilient future.

In the chapters that follow, we'll continue exploring other guideposts for raising emotionally resilient children with DMDD. Building on the foundation of empathy, we'll go on to also include effective communication strategies, problem-solving skills, and the development of self-discipline. While all of these skills are interconnected, empathy is the thread that ties them together and ensures that a child with DMDD can thrive despite their challenges.

Chapter 5
Effective Communication and Listening Actively

Bella and Lizzie's Story

Bella and Lizzie Stein, identical twin girls, faced a challenging journey alongside their family as they coped with DMDD. Their mother Abigail recounted the tumultuous path that began before their birth and continued through their teenage years.

The story begins with a complex and stressful pregnancy. Abigail—who was already caring for four children and working nights—was overwhelmed when she discovered that she was expecting twins. Despite the challenges, however, the pregnancy was relatively uneventful. The girls were delivered via C-section at 36 weeks, weighing 6 pounds, 8 ounces, and 7 pounds, 8 ounces. After a short stay in the NICU for jaundice and low blood sugar, Bella and Lizzie joined the family at home, where they were warmly welcomed.

Abigail recalled, "The first year with the twins was special—Bella and Lizzie were sweet and everyone adored them. However, life became increasingly complicated as they grew more mobile around their first birthday." Unlike their older siblings, Bella and Lizzie were shy and hesitant to warm up to people at church or extended family gatherings. "The first time we really started thinking that something was different about Bella and Lizzie was when we started talking to them about going to kindergarten," said Abigail. "They hadn't attended preschool, which meant that kindergarten would be their first experience with school. Every time we talked to them about it, they would become unhinged, screaming and crying and saying they didn't want to go."

As the twins grew older, their behavior became more concerning. They started showing signs of severe anxiety and depression. Abigail recalled that by third grade, the family was at their wit's end. That prompted them to make an appointment with a child psychiatrist. Thus began a long and complex journey through various diagnoses and treatments. Initially diagnosed with anxiety and depression, Bella and Lizzie were later diagnosed with DMDD. Lizzie also received a diagnosis of selective mutism, and although she seemed to outgrow it, she continued to struggle with speaking in new or frightening situations. Bella, on the other hand, developed a tic disorder and exhibited symptoms of obsessive compulsive disorder. However, the latter was never officially diagnosed.

The twins' behaviors were difficult to manage at home. Abigail recalled, "They would have explosive outbursts that led to holes being punched in walls, doors ripped off hinges, mirrors smashed, and food thrown across the kitchen. Lizzie would often express her frustration through destructive behavior. At the same time, Bella would resort to self-harm, banging her head against the cement floor." These episodes were terrifying and heartbreaking for their parents, who felt utterly helpless. But as you'll learn at the conclusion of this chapter, hope and improvement were not far away.

Reflecting on Communication: A Path to Fostering Resilience in Children

The challenge of communicating with a child with DMDD is a daunting one: parents must simultaneously keep important goals in mind and communicate effectively, free of intense emotions. Of course, when parents are frustrated, they're more vulnerable to bringing excess baggage from the past into current situations. However, the more successful parents become at examining their own goals and motives and questioning whether their communication is advancing them *toward* their goals or inhibiting them from *reaching* their goals, the more effectively parents will be able to communicate and the more they'll be able to foster resilience in their children. To that end, parents might ask themselves several critical questions to ensure that their approach aligns with their objectives for their children's long-term growth and development.

We suggest that parents take a few minutes to consider each of these questions about the importance of how they're communicating and the impact their messages are having on their children.

Questions to Evaluate Communication Practices

Do my messages convey and teach respect?

Respect is foundational to any relationship, and it's essential that parents model respect in their communications with their children *and* with others—children are always listening! For the Morgan family, this meant David and Elena rethinking how they responded to Maya's outbursts. Initially, their frustration often led to harsh words or dismissive attitudes, and that only escalated Maya's anger. David and Elena realized that they needed to change their approach by first asking themselves if their responses were conveying caring and respect for Maya. They began to practice calm, respectful communication even in the heat of the moment, modeling the kind of more sensitive behavior they wanted their daughter to emulate. Over time, this shift helped Maya learn to express her emotions more respectfully, improving their home's overall atmosphere.

Am I fostering realistic expectations in my children?

Setting realistic expectations is crucial in helping children develop a healthy sense of self and resilience. This task is especially challenging for a child with DMDD, as the Guptas discovered with their daughter. They often found themselves pushing Anika to manage her emotions in ways that were beyond her developmental capacity, leading to frustration on both sides. Once they started reflecting on whether or not their expectations were realistic, however, Raj and Priya adjusted their approach—they began setting smaller, more achievable goals for Anika's emotional regulation. During calmer moments, when Anika was more receptive to hearing her parents, Raj and Priya would teach their daughter to take deep breaths or step away for a few minutes when she was feeling overwhelmed. This helped Anika feel more capable and less discouraged when she started feeling agitated and ultimately improved her confidence and resilience.

Am I helping my children learn how to solve problems?

Problem-solving is a critical life skill that can be nurtured through thoughtful communication. The Browns often stepped in to solve problems for Liam, especially when his anxiety made him hesitant to engage with challenges, but they eventually realized that although it made their lives a bit easier to "rescue" Liam, by doing so, they were robbing him of the opportunity to develop his own problem-solving skills. On top of that, they were unintentionally conveying the message to Liam that he wasn't capable of confronting problems. Sarah and Michael recognized that they had to modify their approach. Instead of immediately offering solutions, they started to guide Liam through identifying the problem, considering possible solutions, and evaluating the outcomes. This empowered him to tackle challenges more independently and reduced his overall anxiety as he gained confidence in his problem-solving abilities.

Am I teaching empathy and compassion?

As we noted in the previous chapter, being able to teach children to have empathy and compassion is a crucial component of parenting and one that requires parents to become increasingly attuned to their children's emotional experiences. For the Morgans, this required paying more attention to Maya's experiences and validating her feelings rather than focusing primarily on correcting her behavior. David and Elena realized that they had to improve how they modeled and taught empathy, so they changed their style and began to actively express understanding and compassion during challenging moments. This approach helped Maya feel more understood and less isolated in her struggles and encouraged her to be more empathic toward others, including her younger sibling. Emphasizing empathy can help parents feel more connected to their children's emotional needs.

Am I promoting self-discipline and self-control?

Self-discipline and self-control are essential traits for resilience and success in life. The Guptas, recognizing that Anika struggled with self-control during her emotional outbursts, began to focus on promoting these qualities through consistent routines and clear expectations, and they also helped Anika create a calm-down routine. The one that she favored was hugging a favorite stuffed dog. This strategy was strengthened when Anika began to rub the stuffed animal on her own while also saying "Calm down" in a reassuring way. This routine empowered her to handle her feelings more independently and effectively, plus it provided her with a sense of accomplishment, thus reinforcing her self-discipline.

Am I setting limits that permit my children to learn from me rather than resent me?

Setting limits is a necessary part of parenting, but how those limits are established can significantly affect how they're received. The Browns faced this challenge when trying to set boundaries around Liam's screen time—that often triggered his anxiety. Instead of imposing limits unilaterally, Sarah and Michael started involving Liam in the decision-making process, explaining their reasons and listening to his concerns. They set limits in a collaborative rather than authoritarian way by asking themselves if their approach was likely to teach Liam or make him resentful.

One strategy that worked very effectively was for Sarah and Michael to set certain parameters and then offer Liam some choice within those parameters. For instance, Liam often had assigned homework of about 30 minutes each school day evening. He was given the choice of doing his homework right after having his after-school snack (often the homework was done on the computer, but that didn't count toward his screen time) and then getting to have 30 minutes of screen time for non-homework activities, or he could do those things in the opposite order.

The Browns then allowed Liam an additional 30 minutes of screen time after dinner that had to end at least 30 minutes before going to bed. Not only did this approach reduce Liam's resistance to having limits set for his screen use, it also taught him valuable lessons about selfregulation and the importance of balance. This kind of emphasis on collaborative limit-setting can be helpful in a variety of situations.

Am I truly listening to and validating what my children are saying?

Listening is a fundamental aspect of effective communication, yet it's often overlooked, especially in stressful situations. The Guptas realized they were sometimes so focused on managing Anika's behavior that they weren't truly listening to her. They decided to consciously attempt to give her the space to express herself to be sure that they were genuinely listening and validating Anika's feelings. Rather than immediately yelling at her to stop her behavior—which only added to her frustration and outbursts—they would speak with her in a gentle way, offering such comments as "We can see you're very upset about [whatever made her upset]. We know it's not easy, but once you're able to calm down a little, we can try to figure out what will help the situation." This change in intensity and tone of voice made Anika feel heard and respected, and that in turn made her more receptive to their guidance.

Do my children know that I value their input?

Valuing a child's input fosters a sense of agency and confidence. Similar to what the Guptas did with Anika, the Morgans rethought how they would include Maya in family decisions. They began to actively seek her opinions on matters that affected her, such as weekend activities or family rules. They asked Maya what she thought about a particular rule or how she would like to spend the weekend and then would take her suggestions seriously. Sometimes they would concur with what she recommended; other times, they weren't able to do so. However, whenever the latter occurred, they carefully reviewed the reasons for their decision with Maya, reinforcing the concept that her opinion was valued. Slowly, Maya's cooperation and sense of empowerment increased.

Do my children know how special they are to me?

Children need to feel loved and valued, not just through words but through actions as well. The Browns made it a point to regularly remind Liam of how special he was to them, both during moments of success and during their everyday interactions with him—they integrated small gestures of affection into their days and took time to celebrate Liam's unique qualities. These actions reinforced Liam's sense of self-worth, which played a crucial role in him becoming better able to manage his anxiety.

Am I assisting my children to appreciate that mistakes are part of learning?

Understanding that mistakes are a natural part of learning is essential for developing resilience. Raj and Priya recognized that Anika often became overly upset when she made mistakes—she feared she had disappointed them. By asking themselves whether they were helping Anika see mistakes as learning opportunities, they began to change how they responded to her errors. Instead of expressing disappointment, they would engage Anika in a discussion of what she could learn from the situation, and they also paid special attention to praising her efforts. As a result of these changes, Anika became more resilient and less fearful of making mistakes.

> We learned early that our son would get extremely angry with himself when he made mistakes or got in trouble. He was also embarrassed, and it was common for him to give in to a cascade of negative self-talk such as, "I hate myself. I can't do anything right." To combat these tendencies, we would hug him tightly and talk him through the issue by asking him questions like, "Do other kids at school also make mistakes or get in trouble? What happens to them? Are they okay the next day? You're going to be okay, too." Showing empathy instead of anger when he would get in trouble helped kick him out of the cycle of negative thoughts and feelings about himself.

Am I comfortable with acknowledging my own mistakes and apologizing when it's indicated?

Modeling accountability is a powerful way to teach children the importance of assuming responsibility for their own actions and mistakes. The Morgans realized that they had reacted too harshly to Maya's behavior at some points in the past and that it was necessary to acknowledge those mistakes and learn from them. To that end, David and Elena started to model humility and accountability by asking themselves whether they were comfortable apologizing. When they made a mistake, they would apologize to Maya, showing her that it's okay to admit when you're wrong and that doing so is a strength, not a weakness. They were also careful not to continue to repeat the same mistake again lest their apologies be experienced as hollow and not genuine. This practice strengthened their relationship with Maya and taught her to take responsibility for her actions.

By continually reflecting on these kinds of questions, parents can ensure that their communication strategies are aligned with their long-term goals of fostering resilience, empathy, and self-discipline in their children. These examples from the Morgans, Guptas, and Browns illustrate how thoughtful, reflective communication can transform challenges into opportunities for growth and learning. Effective communication and active listening are foundational skills for fostering resilience in all children and particularly in those diagnosed with DMDD. Children with DMDD often experience intense emotional outbursts and chronic irritability, making it difficult for them to manage their emotions and interact positively with others. This disorder not only challenges the child but also places significant stress on family dynamics as parents and siblings struggle to understand and respond to these intense behaviors. The importance of effective communication in this context cannot be overstated—it serves as a bridge between the child's emotional world and the family's efforts to provide support and guidance.

The journey toward improved communication has been transformative for the three families we've heard from. Each family faced unique challenges related to their child's DMDD, yet all discovered that a critical key to managing their child's behavior was how they communicated with them. Initially, like many parents, these three families approached their children's outbursts with a mix of discipline, reasoning, and attempts to impose control— strategies that are often effective with children who do not have DMDD. However, these approaches frequently backfired, escalating the situation rather than calming it. The parents were left feeling frustrated, helpless, and sometimes defeated.

As these families learned, traditional methods of communication (such as giving instructions or setting boundaries) need to be adapted when dealing with a child with DMDD. The disorder's hallmark symptoms—persistent irritability and frequent, severe temper outbursts—often mean that children are not in a state where they can quickly process information or respond rationally. Thus, effective communication and the tone used when speaking with children with DMDD require shifting from merely transmitting information or enforcing rules to creating a safe, empathic space where the child feels heard and understood.

A first step for these families was to focus on active listening. Active listening involves more than just hearing what the child says—it requires fully engaging with the child's emotional state, listening without judgment, and responding in ways that validate the child's feelings. For example, when Liam experienced an outburst, his parents began practicing active listening by pausing their initial reactions (like offering solutions or reprimanding him) and instead focusing on acknowledging his emotions, saying things like, "I can see you're upset right now." That helped Liam feel understood, which gradually reduced the intensity of his outbursts.

Similarly, Raj and Priya found that Anika was more receptive when they validated her feelings instead of trying to correct her behavior immediately. They learned to respond to her with statements like, "I understand that you're feeling frustrated. Let's try and figure out what we can do." Such responses helped de-escalate situations and opened the door to having more productive conversations later.

The Morgan family also found that by modeling calm behavior and using compassionate language, they could set the tone for more positive interactions with Maya. They recognized that their emotional responses played a significant role in how Maya reacted and they worked to model the emotional regulation they wanted to see in her.

The experiences of the Brown, Gupta, and Morgan families illustrate that effective communication and active listening aren't just beneficial in managing DMDD—they're essential. By prioritizing empathy, validation, and emotional connection over immediate problem-solving or punitive disciplinary measures, these families were able to foster more robust and empathic relationships, which ultimately led to a more peaceful and supportive home environment. This chapter delves deeper into these strategies, offering practical guidance for other families who are facing similar challenges.

The Role of Communication in Managing DMDD

Children with DMDD struggle with emotional regulation, making it difficult for them to express their feelings calmly and constructively. This can lead to frequent and intense outbursts that can strain communication within the family. For Michael and Sarah, their son Liam's explosive reactions often left them feeling helpless and frustrated. They realized that their usual methods of communication—reasoning, setting boundaries—were ineffective in de-escalating his emotional storms. Instead, they needed to develop new communication methods to help Liam feel understood and supported.

Raj and Priya Gupta faced a similar challenge when Anika would shut down emotionally during arguments—their attempts to reason with her only seemed to push her further away. They learned that effectively communicating with a child experiencing DMDD required a shift from trying to "fix" the problem to actively listening and validating their child's feelings, even when those feelings seemed irrational or disproportionate to the situation.

Strategies for Improving Communication

Active Listening: Fully Engaging with Your Child

Active listening involves more than just hearing the words a child is saying—it requires full engagement, understanding, and thoughtful responses. Parents must listen and learn before they can intervene successfully. For the Brown family, this meant giving their son Liam their undivided attention during his emotional verbal outbursts even though those were often difficult and painful to hear. They learned that the key to defusing these intense situations was not to interrupt him when he was having a verbal outburst despite having the instinct to immediately correct him or tell him to calm down. Instead, they practiced letting Liam speak until he had fully expressed his feelings.

At one point, Michael and Sarah questioned whether allowing Liam's verbal outbursts to continue longer than they would have preferred was "giving in" to him. Perhaps he had much more control over his outbursts than they had originally assumed and he was "using" his outbursts in a manipulative way. However, as they became more informed about DMDD, they learned that Liam did *not* have control of his explosive behaviors and that harsh measures on their part would only serve to exacerbate the problem.

Similarly, almost all parents of a child with DMDD have had to modify their approach with that child and treat them differently than how they have treated their other children. When parents do take an alternative approach, it's important to explain the reasons why to their other children in a nonjudgmental way. They've likely had to do the same with family and friends who were inclined to comment on their inconsistencies and their seeming inability to control the behaviors of the child with DMDD.

As Liam's parents attempted to implement their new approach and not immediately jump in with advice, they found the change to be very challenging—listening to Liam's harsh words without reacting was a test of their patience and their own emotional control. However, they soon noticed that by allowing Liam to vent his frustrations fully (as long as it didn't involve destructive behaviors), he gradually became less agitated. Over time, Liam started to feel more secure knowing that he was being heard, which in turn reduced the frequency and intensity of his outbursts.

As one example, when Liam would come home from school upset about something that had happened with a classmate, his parents resisted the urge to immediately offer solutions or downplay his feelings or tell him to calm down. Instead, they listened intently, asking gentle questions like "What happened next?" and "How did that make you feel?" This provided Liam with a safe space to articulate his emotions and it helped him process his feelings more effectively. By practicing active listening, Michael and Sarah helped Liam develop a greater sense of self-awareness and trust in them—he knew that they valued his feelings and opinions no matter how difficult they were for him to express.

Validation: Acknowledging Your Child's Emotions

Validation is about acknowledging and accepting your child's feelings as being genuine and essential even when you don't necessarily agree with their perspective. For Raj and Priya, this approach transformed their relationship with Anika. She had often felt isolated and misunderstood, and her go-to expression had been telling her parents that no one cared about her. In the past, Raj and Priya's immediate reaction was to reassure her by saying, "Of course we care about you!" or to try and correct her by explaining all the ways they showed their care.

However, they realized that this response often left Anika feeling alone and unheard, and so they began to practice validation instead. When Anika expressed these feelings, Raj and Priya stepped back from trying to fix the situation and instead directly acknowledged her emotions, saying, "I can see you're upset right now. It sounds like you feel lonely! Let's talk about what's going on."

This approach didn't mean they agreed with Anika's belief that no one cared about her, but they nonetheless recognized and respected her feelings. By validating her emotions, Raj and Priya opened the door to more meaningful conversations about what was genuinely bothering Anika. She became more willing to discuss her feelings because she knew her parents wouldn't just dismiss them outright. This helped Anika feel more secure and understood, which made her more open to working with her parents to find solutions to her problems.

One evening, after a particularly difficult day at school, Anika came home and tearfully declared that she felt like no one at school liked her. Instead of reassuring her that she was wellliked, Raj asked, "What happened today that made you feel this way?" That simple question allowed Anika to open up about a specific incident with a classmate and led to a deeper discussion about how she could handle such situations in the future. Having her feelings validated made Anika feel valued and helped her build more confidence to face future challenges more effectively.

Setting Boundaries with Compassion: Balancing Limits and Empathy

While validating a child's emotions is crucial, setting clear boundaries is equally important to help them manage their behavior. The Morgan family discovered that setting limits with Maya was most effective when they did so with both calmness and compassion. Maya often had difficulty following instructions, and situations could quickly escalate into a power struggle if they weren't handled carefully.

When Maya had refused to follow a request in the past, her parents had responded with frustration or stern discipline. Both only served to heighten the tension. They learned that a different approach was required, one that combined clear expectations with empathy. For example, when it was time for Maya to set the table—a task she often resisted—her parents would calmly restate the boundary. "Maya, it's time to set the table now," they said, and paired their statement with a choice that allowed Maya to feel some control, such as, "Would you like to do it now, or would you prefer to take five minutes and then do it?"

They also learned another strategy to use when Maya told them that they were "always nagging her"—David and Elena told Maya that sometimes they might forget to do something, too, and if they did forget, they would like Maya to "remind" them by simply telling them what they had forgotten to do. They then asked Maya how she would like them to remind her so that it didn't feel like "nagging."

The fact David and Elena had first told Maya how they would like to be reminded made it easier for Maya to then reply, "Just tell me in a calm voice." Although her parents felt they had always typically used such a voice, they answered, "Thanks for letting us know! We'll make certain we speak calmly in the future." After reaching that agreement, they used a calm voice to remind Maya to do things, and when they did so, she no longer felt like they were nagging since it was her idea of how she wanted to be reminded.

Modeling Emotional Regulation: Teaching by Example

Children often learn to manage their emotions by observing the adults around them. This realization was a turning point for the Brown family in dealing with Liam's intense outbursts— they noticed that their emotional reactions often mirrored Liam's, leading to a cycle of escalating tensions. They recognized the need for change and committed to modeling healthier emotional regulation techniques.

Instead of reacting immediately when Liam's behavior became challenging, they practiced deep breathing and they took a moment to calm themselves before responding. If Liam began shouting in frustration over a homework assignment, rather than immediately correcting him or showing their frustration, his parents took a deep breath and calmly said, "I can see you're upset right now. Let's take a moment to breathe together and then figure this out." This approach required Michael and Sarah to develop more of their own self-awareness and emotional control.

The results were significant! As Liam watched his parents remain calm and composed during his outbursts, he began to imitate their behaviors, and over time, Liam started to adopt those techniques himself: when he felt an outburst coming, he sometimes paused and took a deep breath, a behavior he had learned from watching his parents.

One particular instance stood out when Liam was frustrated because he couldn't find his soccer ball. He was on the verge of a meltdown. Instead of frantically searching for the ball or mirroring his growing distress, Sarah calmly said, "Liam, I can see this is upsetting you. Let's sit down and take a few deep breaths together before we look for it." Surprisingly, Liam followed her lead, and after a few moments of calm breathing, they were able to search for the soccer ball together without Liam's behavior escalating into a full-blown outburst.

By consistently modeling emotional regulation, Michael and Sarah taught Liam that there are constructive ways to handle strong emotions. That lesson didn't just help reduce the frequency and intensity of his outbursts, it equipped Liam with lifelong skills for managing stress and frustration. On top of that, the resulting shift in the family dynamic created a more peaceful home environment that empowered Liam to take better control of his emotional responses.

Finding Solutions to Challenges and Obstacles

Parenting is a journey filled with rewarding moments and significant challenges. While every family strives to maintain open and effective communication, misunderstandings and conflicts are inevitable, especially when dealing with intense emotions, behavioral issues, or a child's unique dynamics. However, by recognizing that setbacks are a natural part of the parenting process and by employing a range of strategies, parents can navigate these challenges effectively, bolstering growth and understanding within the family. The sense of control and empowerment that comes from effectively navigating setbacks can boost parents' confidence and make them feel more capable in their roles.

The Guptas, Browns, and Morgans faced distinct challenges in their parenting journeys. Their stories provide valuable insights into how parents can approach difficulties with empathy, discipline, consistency, and a focus on long-term growth while addressing the obstacles that hinder effective communication.

Understanding the nature of setbacks is the first step in addressing parenting challenges. Setbacks are inevitable and should not be viewed as failures! Instead, they are opportunities for growth and learning. For the Guptas, there were moments when their daughter's emotional outbursts were overwhelming. Despite their best efforts at active listening and validation, at times, these communication skills did not seem to be effective. During such moments, Raj and Priya realized the importance of patience. They gave Anika the space she needed to process her emotions. They began to see challenging moments as learning opportunities rather than failures. After difficult episodes, they would self-reflect, considering their responses and evaluating what had worked and what didn't. These periods of reflection and the sense of growth and learning they brought helped Raj and Priya approach future situations with more understanding and patience. This process can make all parents feel more knowledgeable and insightful in their parenting journeys.

The Guptas' experience highlights the importance of providing a child space when emotions are high. When Anika's outbursts peaked, her parents found that stepping back and allowing her to calm down independently was more effective than jumping in and attempting to resolve the issue immediately. Then, after Anika had had time to settle down, they would have a calm and constructive conversation with her about what had happened. This approach helped Anika feel more in control of her emotions and strengthened her trust in her parents—she knew that they respected her need for space.

A period of calming down allows for blood to flow back to a child's prefrontal cortex, heightening their ability to reason and rationalize. In contrast, when intense emotional dysregulation turns into rage, it's not unusual for a child to not even remember what has taken place—that's one reason why attempting to process a meltdown with a child who may not even recall what occurred is typically futile.

One of the recurring challenges for the Browns involved Liam's homework—he often struggled with his assignments (particularly in math), prompting his anxiety to flare up. Then whenever Sarah or Michael tried to help, he would interpret their guidance as criticism and become defensive and frustrated. That led to tense standoffs during which Liam shut down completely and refused to continue. The Browns, wanting to support their son, sometimes pushed harder and tried to explain the concepts again, but their efforts only worsened the situation. Liam often ended up in tears, feeling misunderstood and overwhelmed.

Over time, Michael and Sarah realized that they were unintentionally heightening Liam's anxiety. They learned to shift their communication style—they let Liam know that they were available to help whenever he asked them for assistance but didn't attempt to immediately step in. They also encouraged him to take breaks when they noticed him becoming stressed. Instead of focusing solely on completing the homework, they emphasized the process of focusing on it, praising Liam for his efforts rather than the outcome. This change in communication helped reduce his tension around homework and permitted Liam to approach his assignments with less fear and more confidence.

For the Morgan family, the challenge was to use empathy to guide their disciplinary practices, especially when Maya became physically aggressive. David and Elena recognized that they needed to understand and address the underlying causes of their daughter's behavior, but they also knew that their first priority was to enforce clear boundaries to ensure her safety and the safety of others. They recognized that they had to carry out their disciplinary practices with as much empathy as possible—they needed to ensure that Maya understood why her behavior was unacceptable without feeling overly shamed. They accomplished this by explaining to Maya why her behavior wasn't acceptable and how it affected others while also reassuring her that they still loved her and were there to help her learn from her mistakes.

> At age six, my daughter disliked wearing her coat even when it was freezing outside. As I headed out to the car with several bags, I asked my daughter if she wanted to wear her coat to school or carry it instead. She quickly said, "Carry it!" So, she picked up her coat and carried it to the car. It mattered little to me if she wore it. My goal was for her to take it to school with her. Providing her options to wear her coat or carry was a win-win for both of us.

To improve their parenting skills, David and Elena also sought out therapeutic support. The therapist provided them with strategies tailored to Maya's needs and helped them create a plan that combined immediate consequences with follow-up discussions. This allowed Maya to begin to understand the impacts of her actions while also addressing the emotions that led to her behavior. As Maya felt more secure with the establishment of clear and consistent routines, her outbursts lessened; she knew that there was a framework for addressing issues whenever they arose. If she hit her younger sibling, for example, the consequence might be a brief time-out followed by a conversation about what had happened. By combining immediate consequences with an empathic follow-up discussion, the Morgans helped Maya learn from her mistakes without feeling shamed or rejected.

Consistency is a critical factor in effective parenting—children thrive in environments where they know what to expect, and consistent responses from parents help build this sense of security. But consistency shouldn't be mistaken for rigidity! Parents must remain adaptable and recognize that different situations may require different approaches. Even when Anika's outbursts were challenging, for example, her parents consistently provided her with space to calm down and then followed that with a debriefing session. This approach helped Anika feel secure and strengthened her emotional regulation skills.

The Morgans also balanced consistency with adaptability. As Maya grew older, her needs and the nature of her challenges changed, so although David and Elena continued to consistently enforce consequences for aggressive behavior, they also adapted their approach as Maya's emotional intelligence developed. This flexibility helped Maya continue to learn and grow.

The experiences of both the Gupta and Morgan families underscore that successful parenting involves striking a delicate balance between empathy, discipline, consistency, and adaptability while embracing inevitable setbacks and seeing them as opportunities for growth.

One of the most significant obstacles in communicating with children who have DMDD is the heightened emotional states that both the child and the parents often find themselves in during a crisis. In the Morgan household, David and Elena struggled to maintain calm during Maya's outbursts—their initial reactions were usually defensive or dismissive, which only intensified Maya's anger and frustration. They found that their emotional responses were a barrier to effective communication as they were often too overwhelmed to listen actively or respond empathically.

Another obstacle is the tendency to focus on the child's behavior rather than the underlying emotions driving the behavior. The Guptas often met Anika's outbursts with attempts to correct her behavior through punitive discipline, a strategy that failed to address the root cause of her distress. They had to learn to look beyond the surface behavior and focus on what Anika was trying to communicate through her actions.

For the Browns, a significant communication barrier arose whenever Michael and Sarah discussed any plans or changes in routine, such as vacations or weekend activities. Liam often had trouble articulating his feelings, especially when he was anxious about a new experience, so when his parents excitedly talked about an upcoming trip, Liam would withdraw, becoming quiet and unresponsive. Sarah and Michael initially misinterpreted his silence as disinterest or defiance and would get frustrated. They would attempt to coax Liam into participating in the conversation, but their insistence would only make him retreat further. The end result was a breakdown in communication. It wasn't until they deeply understood that Liam's withdrawal was a sign of anxiety rather than disinterest that they adjusted their approach.

Instead of pressing him to engage, they gave Liam more time to process the information and express his feelings at his own pace. They also began checking in with him one-on-one, allowing him to share his concerns in a lower-pressure environment. Their new approach helped Liam feel more understood and allowed Michael and Sarah to address his anxieties before they became overwhelming, leading to more effective communication within the family.

Despite their respective obstacles, all three families improved their communication style and their understanding of their children's needs. The Morgans learned to recognize their own emotional triggers and worked on maintaining calm during Maya's outbursts, a tactic that allowed them to respond more effectively. The Guptas shifted their focus from merely correcting Anika's behavior to understanding the emotions driving it, which led to more meaningful conversations and better outcomes for their daughter. Similarly, the Browns discovered that when they gave Liam space to process his emotions and addressed his anxiety with patience and understanding, they could better support his needs and reduce his stress.

While every family strives to maintain open and effective communication, misunderstandings and conflicts are of course inevitable. However, by recognizing that setbacks are a natural part of the parenting process and employing a range of strategies, parents can navigate these challenges effectively, fostering growth and understanding within the family.

> My son's D3 level was low, and I couldn't understand why since I gave him Vitamin D3 daily. When I read that oxcarbazepine can lower D3 levels and interfere with absorption, I started to give him Vitamin D3 hours after his morning medication. However, the game changer was when I learned that K2 and magnesium in proper proportion are essential to maximize Vitamin D3 absorption. That is when my son's D3 levels reached optimal levels. I also give him omega-3 fatty acids to support his ADHD, as it may help with cognitive focus, and decreasing inflammation.

Returning to the Twins

School became increasingly problematic for Bella and Lizzie. Their anxiety and aversion to school worsened, leading to frequent absences and them falling behind academically. But despite these challenges, their behavior at school was reported as being generally positive, which puzzled their parents. Their middle school counselor suggested that the girls were "bottling up their emotions" throughout the school day, only to explode when they returned home to their "safe space."

The situation reached a critical point when the twins were 12 years old. Lizzie required inpatient hospitalization, marking the first time they were separated. During this period, their parents realized that the girls were each other's biggest triggers—Bella's behavior improved significantly while Lizzie was away. To help manage the situation at home, the family decided to give each twin their own bedroom, which involved converting the family room into a makeshift bedroom for their older brother. This adjustment helped reduce the escalations between Bella and Lizzie, although it did place additional strain on their neurotypical siblings.

The twins also encountered the police and Child Protective Services (CPS) representatives. On one occasion, after a fight with their older sister, Bella and Lizzie ran to a neighbor's house. The startled neighbor called the police. Another incident involved Lizzie threatening to jump out of a moving car, prompting Abigail to pull over and call 911.

Abigail recounted the difficult times that had required outside intervention. "We had multiple visits from our local police department and had to stand by helplessly as they entered our home," she explained. "These visits would involve breaking interior doors off their hinges, tackling the girls, pinning them down, handcuffing them or strapping them to stretchers, and hauling them off to hospitals and police stations."

In a desperate attempt to find stability, Abigail explored Dr. Matthews' DMDD protocol. The twins' providers were unfamiliar with it and hesitant to try it, so Abigail found a different doctor who knew a little about the protocol and *was* willing to try it. "During that time, we were planning a move across country to be nearer to a residential treatment center for Lizzie," said Abigail. "Though that had been a heartbreaking decision for us to make, we felt like we had no other choice by that point." But as the family was getting closer to moving and the girls were titrating up on the protocol medications, glimmers of stability emerged, and when they finally reached their destination, it was evident that the medications were having a positive effect on both daughters.

The twins' behavior began to improve significantly—they had fewer outbursts and were experiencing a more regulated emotional state. Consequently, the family didn't have to put Lizzie into a residential setting. Instead, they were able to stay together as a family and start life in a new state.

Conclusion: Building Stronger Family Connections

Effective communication is the cornerstone of a resilient family dynamic, especially when managing a complex condition like DMDD. For families likes the Browns, Guptas, and Morgans, the path to improving communication was marked by learning, adapting, and growing together. Through consistent practice and a deep commitment to understanding their children's unique needs, these families were able to foster stronger, more empathic relationships, creating a foundation of resilience that supported every family member.

For Michael and Sarah, active listening became the key to unlocking deeper connections with their son Liam. They created an environment where he eventually felt safe to express his feelings without fear of judgment. Achieving that new atmosphere wasn't easy—the Browns had to suppress their instincts to immediately correct or comfort and instead focus on the reasons for Liam's behavior. Over time, as Liam realized that his parents genuinely wanted to understand his emotions, the intensity and frequency of his outbursts began to decrease.

For the Gupta family, validation was the turning point in their relationship with Anika. Whenever Anika expressed loneliness and neglect, Raj and Priya learned the power of acknowledging her emotions without immediately trying to fix them. This shift from correcting Anika's feelings to validating them opened the door to more honest and constructive conversations. Anika began to feel more understood and supported, which made her more willing to discuss her struggles and work collaboratively with her parents to find solutions. Validation didn't just improve communication, it strengthened the trust and emotional bonds between Anika and her parents.

Meanwhile, the Morgan family discovered the importance of setting compassionate boundaries, particularly when managing Maya's behavioral challenges. They realized that punitive discipline alone was ineffective and that they needed to be empathetic when setting boundaries. They were able to reduce the incidences of power struggles by calmly restating their expectations and offering Maya different options for completing a task. This helped her feel respected and involved in the decision-making process. As a result, Maya began to adhere to the boundaries her parents set. The new family dynamics gave her a sense of improved autonomy and control within a structured environment.

For all of these families, modeling emotional regulation was another critical strategy that transformed their family dynamics. The Browns found that by managing their emotional reactions, they could better guide Liam in handling his own emotions. This process of selfregulation, of parents consciously practicing calming techniques before responding to their children, became a powerful model for their children to emulate. As the parents became more adept at managing their own emotions, their children began to mirror their behaviors, leading to fewer emotional outbursts and a more peaceful home environment.

These strategies—active listening, validation, compassionate boundary-setting, and modeling emotional regulation—are not quick fixes. They require time, patience, and consistent practice. However, as these families discovered, the rewards can be profound. By focusing on these particular communication techniques, the parents improved their children's behavior and strengthened their overall family dynamics. They learned that the key to effective communication doesn't lie in eliminating all conflicts but rather in navigating them with patience, understanding, and a shared commitment to working through challenges together.

Building stronger family connections in the face of DMDD is a journey, not a destination. It involves continuous effort and the willingness to grow together as a family. But through effective communication, families can foster an environment where every member feels heard, valued, and supported—in the process creating a resilient family dynamic that can weather even the most challenging storms. The experiences of the Browns, Guptas, and Morgans serve as a testament to the power of communication in transforming relationships and nurturing a deep sense of connection and resilience.

Chapter 6
Accepting Our Children for Who They Are: Conveying Unconditional Love and Setting Realistic Expectations

Barry's Story

Barry's story began when the O'Learys adopted him when he was a drug-exposed infant. His early exposure brought struggles with temperament and sleep. Then as a young child, he started experiencing rages that prompted his mother Carol to use restraint techniques she had learned during foster parenting classes; those techniques were designed to prevent him from harming himself or others. But his rages escalated as he grew, with Barry becoming increasingly irritable and explosive and triggered by the most minor of frustrations. This interracial family described living in constant fear of their son.

"He was in second grade and about the same size as me," Carol said. During that year, Barry was diagnosed with ADHD and placed on a stimulant medication. It helped for a few years, but it became ineffective as he reached puberty, so his medication was switched to aripiprazole (Abilify®), a commonly prescribed antipsychotic that also initially helped. However, that also soon lost its effectiveness, and Barry began to experience increased irritability, weight gain, and physical changes.

Carol observed, "My son became obese and developed breasts, and the rages continued. He was miserable. I dreaded picking him up from school every day—he was cranky all the time and nothing could soothe him. But worst of all were the rages, when the littlest thing would set him off. His eyes would get red, he would huff and puff, he would break things and get right up into our faces, he would curse and yell and scream and threaten. It was like being in an abusive relationship where you're walking on eggshells, holding your breath, and trying everything you can think of to fend off the next incident. And when your child is a very dark-skinned, black male who weighs 230 pounds, you fear for his safety as well as your own."

When Carol told her son's psychiatrist what Barry looked like when he was enraged and that then he would collapse and not remember any of it, the psychiatrist told her that what she was describing sounded exactly like a particle seizure. He suspected DMDD, and when Carol mentioned what she'd learned from a parent in an online support group, the psychiatrist began exploring the protocol developed by Dr. Matthews. Despite initial skepticism from their doctor— who was unfamiliar with DMDD—Barry was eventually placed on the protocol.

The treatment marked a turning point for Barry. His constant irritability and explosive rages diminished, allowing him to function more normally. Although Barry still faces challenges related to other diagnoses, the improvements the Matthews Protocol has brought have provided peace at home and hope for his future. Now, instead of seeming to be destined for a life of escalating crises, Barry shows signs of development and functionality, providing both him and his family with a sense of relief and optimism.

In this chapter, we'll explore the transformative power that unconditional love and acceptance play in the growth and development of children, especially those with DMDD. The core message of this chapter is that providing a foundation of unwavering love and acceptance is crucial *and* empowering for parents. Doing so fosters a child's sense of self-worth and their sense of security, both of which are vital for their emotional well-being and personal growth.

The Importance of Unconditional Love

Unconditional love is the foundation of emotional development, especially for children who face challenges such as DMDD. Because of how they struggle to regulate their emotions, they experience intense mood swings and behavioral outbursts. In this context, unconditional love becomes a source of comfort and a stabilizing force, offering a sense of safety amid emotional turbulence.

Children with DMDD can experience overwhelming emotions that they find challenging to manage; such scenarios often lead to frustration, anger, and sadness. This constant cycle of intense feelings can be exhausting and isolating, leaving them feeling misunderstood or unsupported. However, when caregivers respond with unconditional love, it helps ease the children's emotional burden. The reassurance that they're loved even when they're displaying very challenging behaviors helps them feel secure and provides a stable foundation that these children can use to learn how to navigate their emotions over time.

Researchers have consistently demonstrated that children who feel loved and accepted tend to exhibit stronger emotional resilience and a more remarkable ability to manage stress. The impact of this loving foundation cannot be overstated! It helps children develop healthier coping mechanisms and reduces the frequency of emotional outbursts. Knowing that they're loved and accepted even in their most difficult moments can be life-changing for children like Liam, providing the stability they need to thrive.

At first, Liam's parents were overwhelmed by the frequent emotional outbursts that were dominating their daily lives. These intense episodes often left them feeling helpless and unsure about how to respond effectively. They initially focused on controlling Liam's behavior, anticipating his next outburst and trying to prevent it before it spiraled out of control. However, that method only seemed to fuel his emotional storms, increasing tension in the household. Michael and Sarah constantly felt like they were walking on eggshells—they feared that any wrong move could trigger another episode.

The turning point came when they realized that they needed to focus on simply being present instead of controlling emotions. During Liam's difficult moments, they communicated love and acceptance by offering him their unconditional support and reassurance. Sitting with him through the emotional storms without judgment allowed Liam to feel safe and understood. This gradual shift in Michael and Sarah's approach led to a noticeable decrease in the intensity and frequency of Liam's outbursts, helping the family find a new sense of calm and connection.

But a caveat: unconditional love does *not* mean allowing a child to act without consequences or boundaries. It is not permissiveness—rather, unconditional love is an acknowledgment of the child's inherent worth, separate from their behavior. Children with DMDD often feel like they're constantly losing control, and for them, unconditional love provides a stabilizing force: it tells them that no matter how intense their emotions become, they are still valued and cared for. This creates a sense of safety that allows them to navigate their emotional world more confidently.

Demonstrating Unconditional Love

Demonstrating unconditional love goes beyond simply saying "I love you." It involves concrete actions that consistently reinforce the message and help the child feel supported even during challenging moments. For parents of children with DMDD, such actions can feel overwhelming, but the following strategies offer practical ways to show unconditional love:

> We constantly celebrate the small wins throughout our day when most parents of neurotypical children would take those things for granted. My husband and I recognize the small wins, like when we get our son to do a chore when he'd rather be doing something else or noticing when he accepts us telling him, "No," to a specific request without an argument. These small wins motivate us to stay consistent, especially during challenging moments. No matter the task, we find the positives and praise our son so he knows we are proud of him for trying. We can continue to build our son's self-esteem, confidence, and resilience by pointing out these big and small wins.

Consistent Emotional Support

One of the most important ways to display unconditional love is through consistent emotional support. This is especially true for children who face challenges such as DMDD. These children often struggle to regulate their emotions, leading to intense mood swings and behavioral outbursts. In this context, unconditional love becomes a source of comfort and a stabilizing force, offering a sense of safety amid emotional turbulence.

Knowing that they are loved and accepted even in their most difficult moments can be life-changing for children like Liam—this knowledge provides them with the stability they need to thrive. Unconditional love means being available to a child during their emotional highs and lows without judgment. For children who experience emotional storms that seem to emerge out of nowhere, consistent emotional support is a lifeline. When Liam would have one of his outbursts, for example, his parents learned not to try to fix the situation immediately. Instead, they offered him the steady presence he needed, letting him know that they were there for him no matter how big or scary his emotions felt.

The Brown family's journey toward offering consistent emotional support wasn't easy. At first, Michael and Sarah were urged to provide solutions or tell Liam to calm down, but those approaches only made him feel more misunderstood. They later learned that simply being present—holding his hand, rubbing his back—was far more effective. Over time, Liam started to feel more grounded, knowing that his parents were a safe emotional harbor.

Raj and Priya faced similar challenges with Anika, who struggled with mood swings that left her feeling out of control. They too learned the value of consistent emotional support, which they demonstrated by sitting with her during her emotional episodes. Similar to what the Browns did, they focused on simply being present instead of trying to talk her out of her feelings or rushing to fix the problem. Raj would often sit beside Anika quietly, sometimes holding her hand or offering a gentle touch on her shoulder. Priya also adopted this approach, and over time, Anika began to calm down more quickly during her emotional storms because she felt safe and supported. Raj and Priya's message was simple but profound: "We're here and we love you no matter what."

Expressing Affection Through Nonverbal Cues

In moments when words fail or emotions are running too high, nonverbal communication becomes a powerful tool. Physical gestures such as a hug, a gentle hand on the back, or a warm smile can convey more than words ever could. David and Elena discovered that Maya responded better to these quiet, loving gestures than to verbal reassurances alone. After difficult days, instead of focusing on the events that had gone wrong or Maya's frequent anger outbursts, her parents made a habit of ending the day with a hug and a kiss goodnight, followed by the words "We love you."

For Maya, these simple gestures helped her internalize that her worth wasn't tied to how well she had managed her emotions that day. She began to feel more secure in her parents' love, and over time, the intensity of her angry outbursts lessened. The Morgans realized that by using nonverbal affection, they were reinforcing their unconditional love in a way that Maya could more easily understand and accept even when words might feel too overwhelming.

The Gupta family also relied on nonverbal affection to communicate their unconditional love to Anika. During particularly tough days, when Anika's moods were unpredictable and intense, Raj and Priya found that just sitting beside her quietly and holding her hand or offering a gentle touch on her shoulder spoke volumes. Anika didn't always have the words to express her emotions, but the physical presence of her parents provided her with the reassurance she needed. Over time, this consistent nonverbal communication helped Anika feel more comforted and secure—she knew that her parents were there for her even when she felt lost in her emotions.

Reassurance and Validation of Emotions

Reassuring children that their emotions are valid and that they're loved regardless of their behavior is another powerful way to demonstrate unconditional love. The Brown family learned this lesson when Liam's outbursts would spiral out of control, overwhelming everyone in the household. Instead of reacting to the moment's chaos, Michael and Sarah told Liam, "We love you. We know this is hard for you, and we're here to help." Although this reassurance didn't stop the outbursts immediately, it slowly helped Liam feel more understood and less alone in his emotional struggles.

For the Gupta family, validating Anika's emotions became crucial to their approach. Anika often felt misunderstood when her emotions ran high, and that only fueled her frustration. Raj and Priya learned that instead of trying to calm her down or fix the problem immediately, they could say, "We understand that this is hard for you right now." Acknowledging her emotional experience helped Anika feel seen and heard, which eventually allowed her to start calming down on her own. As we emphasized in Chap. 5, the power of validation helped forge a bridge of understanding between Anika and her parents, fostering a deeper connection.

Creating Safe, Predictable Routines

Children with DMDD often thrive when they know what to expect. Creating a predictable routine gives them a sense of control and security, which in turn helps reduce their anxiety and emotional volatility. The Morgan family discovered this when they implemented a more structured daily routine for Maya. They found that by clearly outlining what each day would look like—whether it was school, homework, or playtime—Maya felt more in control of her environment. Predictability helped Maya transition between activities with less emotional fallout and her overall mood became more stable.

Similarly, the Gupta family recognized that transitions were particularly challenging for Anika. Raj and Priya began using a visual schedule to help her see what was coming next in her day, giving her time to prepare for mental changes. This minor adjustment reduced Anika's anxiety and helped her deal with transitions more smoothly.

Spending Quality One-on-One Time Together

One-on-one time with a child who has DMDD is crucial for reinforcing their sense of worth and belonging. For children like Maya and Liam who often feel misunderstood or overwhelmed by their emotions, carving out a particular time that isn't focused on correcting behavior can be deeply healing. The Morgan family made it a point to spend dedicated time with Maya outside of emotionally charged situations—they would walk together, play board games, or chat about her day. Such moments free of the pressure of managing emotions or solving problems allowed Maya to feel connected to her parents in a more positive way.

The Brown family also embraced the importance of one-on-one time. Michael started taking Liam out for short father-and-son activities, like going to the park or having ice cream. These outings had no agenda other than to spend time together, and this helped rebuild the trust and connection that Liam's emotional outbursts had strained. Liam began to look forward to these outings, knowing they involved a space and time where he could be himself without fearing that he would disappoint his parents.

Setting Realistic Expectations

One of the most significant challenges for parents of children with DMDD is setting expectations that are realistic and attainable for their child's unique abilities. *Un*realistic expectations can lead to frustration and disappointment, creating conflict and emotional distress for both the child and the family, whereas setting achievable goals based on the child's strengths and limitations can foster a sense of accomplishment and self-worth. This approach reduces stress and helps nurture resilience, reinforcing the child's capacity to manage their emotions and develop healthier behaviors over time.

Adjusting Expectations with Compassion

Parents often feel societal pressure to push their children to achieve, which can lead to unrealistic expectations. The Morgan family struggled with this when they initially expected Maya to manage her anger and behave like other children her age. When Maya repeatedly failed to meet their expectations, that frustrated her and her parents. The turning point came when the Morgans realized they needed to adjust their expectations to match Maya's capabilities. Instead of expecting her to handle multiple tasks simultaneously, they broke things down into smaller, more manageable steps. Doing so allowed Maya to experience success in areas she could handle, and this progress gradually improved her behavior and self-esteem.

The Brown family also had to adjust their expectations for Liam. Initially, Michael and Sarah wanted Liam to manage his emotions in social settings without causing a scene, but they soon realized that expecting him to remain calm in every situation was unrealistic given his struggles with DMDD. Adjusting their expectations and focusing on smaller, more achievable goals—like helping Liam manage one emotion at a time—allowed him to succeed in ways that felt attainable. This compassionate approach helped reduce the tension between Liam and his parents, creating a more favorable environment for emotional growth.

Breaking Down Larger Goals into Smaller Steps

Breaking down larger goals into smaller, manageable tasks is another effective way to set realistic expectations. For example, the Gupta family found that Anika struggled with schoolwork, especially when she was asked to complete several assignments simultaneously. Raj and Priya decided to break her assignments into smaller tasks, allowing Anika to focus on one thing at a time. Setting achievable mini-goals helped her feel more successful and less overwhelmed. This approach also gave Anika the confidence to tackle larger tasks as she experienced herself making progress bit by bit.

Maya's parents likewise introduced a strategy for her that was similar to what Anika's parents used to help her with transitions. Instead of expecting Maya to shift gears smoothly from one activity to the next, they broke each transition into smaller steps. For instance, when moving from playtime to homework, they would first give Maya a five-minute heads-up and then help her tidy up her toys before gently guiding her to her homework station. This gradual approach reduced Maya's transition resistance and helped her shift to a new activity.

Modeling Flexibility in Expectations

Life is unpredictable, and teaching children to be flexible while maintaining a sense of security is valuable. The Brown family faced this challenge when unexpected changes in plans would often trigger Liam's emotional outbursts. To help Liam learn flexibility, Michael and Sarah began modeling how to adapt to changing circumstances with calmness and reassurance— whenever plans changed, they would calmly explain the change to Liam and offer him choices within the new situation. Over time, as he witnessed his parents handling changes without any signs of panic, this approach helped Liam become more adaptable.

The Gupta family also practiced modeling flexibility for Anika, who struggled with changes in her routine. When unforeseen changes occurred, such as a canceled playdate or a delay in dinner plans, Raj and Priya used those moments as teaching opportunities. Instead of focusing on the disruption, they focused on what could still be enjoyed—for example, if a planned activity was canceled, they would offer Anika choices, like watching a favorite movie or engaging in a fun home activity. This helped Anika see that while life can be unpredictable, it doesn't have to be distressing if you approach it with a flexible mindset.

Encouraging Effort Over Outcome

For children with DMDD, focusing on the process rather than the outcome can relieve pressure and encourage persistence. The Morgan family made this shift with Maya to help her manage her emotions—instead of focusing on whether or not she could avoid an outburst, they praised her for trying to regulate her emotions. "We're so proud of how hard you worked to calm down," they would say, even if the situation didn't resolve perfectly. This focus on effort helped Maya feel supported and motivated to persist because she knew that her parents recognized her hard work rather than expected her to be perfect.

Michael and Sarah adopted this approach with Liam, too—instead of focusing on whether or not he completed an activity perfectly, they emphasized the importance of trying his best. When Liam struggled with a school project, Michael and Sarah praised him for his effort, saying, "We're proud of how much time and energy you put into this." Focusing on effort rather than results helped Liam develop a sense of pride in his work and reduced his anxiety about meeting what he experienced as unrealistic expectations.

Celebrating Strengths

Recognizing and celebrating a child's strengths can significantly boost their confidence and self-worth, particularly in the case of children with DMDD, who often feel overshadowed by their emotional struggles. Highlighting their achievements, no matter how small, creates opportunities to focus on their potential rather than their challenges. Parents and caregivers can shift the narrative from constant correction and criticism to encouragement and positive reinforcement by emphasizing talents, unique abilities, and moments of success. This approach helps children see themselves as capable and valued, giving them more resilience and motivation to persevere through difficulties and ultimately strengthening the parent-child relationship.

Identifying and Reinforcing Strengths

Every child has unique strengths that parents must identify and nurture. The Brown family discovered Liam's talent for drawing when they decided to focus on his strengths rather than his emotional outbursts. By encouraging him to spend time on his artwork, they gave Liam an outlet to express himself creatively. Over time, his self-esteem grew as he saw that his family valued and appreciated his talent. His artwork became a source of pride and a way for him to manage his emotions constructively.

Similarly, the Gupta family noticed that Anika had a special connection with animals— despite her emotional struggles, her empathy for animals was undeniable. Raj and Priya encouraged that trait by allowing Anika to spend time volunteering at a local animal shelter. This opportunity gave Anika a sense of purpose and allowed her to channel her emotions into something positive. Eventually, her work with animals helped build her self-esteem; the positive reinforcement she kept getting from her parents motivated her to continue developing this talent.

> Our son has a special affinity towards animals and would handle them gently and carefully. We also found that holding or hugging an animal when he was upset had the uncanny ability to change his mood immediately and would even prevent a looming meltdown. That is when we adopted his "emotional support rabbit." Anytime he was extremely frustrated, sad, and wanted to fight or run, he learned to go to his rabbit and rock him in the rocking chair. The act of hugging his rabbit was magical, and he quickly calmed down and forgot why he was upset in the first place.

Offering Opportunities to Shine in Their Strengths

Creating opportunities for children to showcase their strengths is essential when it comes to bolstering their self-esteem. The Morgan family encouraged Maya to use her love for storytelling to express herself, allowing her to write and to share her stories with the family. Her storytelling skills helped her feel valued for something other than her ability to control her emotions. Maya began to take pride in her stories, and her sense of worth was reinforced by her parents' encouragement.

For Liam, his artwork also became a way for him to shine. Michael and Sarah made it a point to display his drawings around the house and even encouraged him to enter local art competitions. Their support boosted Liam's confidence and provided him with a constructive outlet for his emotions. The Brown family helped him develop a more positive self-image by focusing on what he did well rather than constantly addressing his struggles.

Compassionately Addressing Difficulties

While celebrating strengths is essential, addressing challenges with empathy and compassion is equally important. Children with DMDD often engage in frustrating behaviors, such as temper outbursts, irritability, and defiance—all of which can strain the parent-child relationship—and focusing solely on correcting these behaviors can lead to a negative cycle of criticism and frustration, a scenario that may further escalate the child's emotional reactions. However, approaching these difficulties with empathy instead of recriminations can create a more supportive and nurturing environment for growth.

Liam's parents initially responded to his frequent emotional outbursts with strict rules and consequences, believing that this would help control his behavior. Unfortunately, their emphasis on control led to increased tension in the household, as Liam felt even more misunderstood and isolated. Gradually, his parents shifted their approach to one rooted in empathy, where they acknowledged Liam's emotional challenges and worked to validate his feelings. This produced noticeable improvements: Liam's outbursts became less intense and he responded more positively to calm, empathic discussions.

For their part, the Morgans also began to respond to Maya compassionately instead of punitively. Rather than relying solely on punishment whenever she had a tantrum, they started using a compassionate approach, offering her a safe space to express her emotions without fear of immediate reprimand. Gradually, Maya began to exhibit better emotional regulation, knowing that her feelings were being heard and understood.

In these examples, shifting from a punitive approach to one based on empathy and unconditional love helped both Liam and Maya feel more supported. This created an increasingly positive parent-child dynamic and reduced the frequency and intensity of the children's disruptive behaviors. The lesson is clear: compassionate parenting not only strengthens the parent-child relationship but also promotes long-term emotional growth and resilience in children with DMDD.

Exploring the Root Cause of Behavior

Understanding the root cause of a child's behavior can contribute to more effective solutions than simply reacting to the behavior itself. The Morgan family realized that Maya's sensory overload often triggered her anger outbursts, so rather than punishing her for her outbursts, they began addressing the underlying issue by creating a calmer, quieter environment whenever they noticed Maya getting overstimulated. David and Elena took into account places outside the home that could be potentially triggering, like a restaurant or a store, and were prepared to lessen their daughter's sensory overload with headphones. This strategy reduced the frequency of her outbursts and gave her the tools to manage her emotions better.

The Brown family also learned to look beyond Liam's behavior to understand what was driving his emotional storms, and they discovered that his outbursts were often prompted when he felt overwhelmed in social situations. By acknowledging this and working with Liam to develop strategies for managing his emotions in such settings, Michael and Sarah were able to help Liam feel more in control of his feelings, thus reducing the frequency and intensity of his outbursts.

Using Reflective Listening

Reflective listening—where parents mirror their child's feelings—is valuable for helping children feel understood and accepted. The Gupta family found this approach to be helpful with Anika, especially when she struggled to articulate her emotions. By repeating what they heard her say (i.e., "It sounds like you're feeling upset because things didn't go how you expected"), Raj and Priya helped Anika feel validated. This reflective listening calmed Anika and opened the door for more constructive conversations about how to handle her emotions in the future.

The Morgan family also found reflective listening to be effective with Maya. Whenever she became anxious about an upcoming school presentation, her parents reflected her feelings by saying, "It sounds like you're feeling nervous because you're worried about speaking in front of the class." By mirroring Maya's emotions, Elena and David helped her feel understood, which eased her anxiety.

Fostering a Supportive Environment

The ultimate goal of unconditional love, acceptance, and realistic expectations is to create a supportive environment where children feel safe expressing their emotions, taking risks, and making mistakes without fear of rejection. This environment fosters a child's sense of security and encourages them to approach challenges with optimism and confidence. For children with DMDD, feeling understood and accepted by their families forms the basic foundation they need to cope with their intense emotions and behaviors.

The Brown family's journey in creating a supportive atmosphere for Liam was guided by understanding and acceptance. Sarah and Michael initially struggled with their expectations of Liam's behavior, especially when he had emotional outbursts in public. They felt embarrassed and pressured to correct his behavior immediately, reactions that often escalated his emotions. However, as they learned more about

DMDD and understood Liam's triggers, they shifted what they were doing. Instead of reprimanding Liam for his outbursts, they began to validate his emotions, acknowledging that they understood why he would be frustrated even if his behavior seemed out of proportion to the situation. By saying things like, "I can see you're really upset right now, and that's okay," they helped Liam feel safe. This shift allowed him to express his emotions without feeling judged, which eventually significantly reduced the frequency of his meltdowns.

Similarly, the Gupta family created a supportive environment for Anika by adjusting their expectations around her schoolwork. Raj and Priya initially had expected Anika to follow a strict homework routine, an expectation that frequently triggered emotional breakdowns when she found the tasks to be overwhelming. Recognizing that this approach wasn't working, they adjusted their expectations and took a more flexible approach—instead of pushing Anika to finish all of her assignments in one sitting, they allowed her to take breaks when she needed to, and also they praised her efforts regardless of whether she completed everything perfectly. Their new approach reduced her anxiety and helped her feel more confident about tackling her schoolwork.

In both families, creating a supportive environment was a pivotal factor in their children's emotional development. By recognizing their children's unique emotional needs and prioritizing love and acceptance over perfection, the Browns and Guptas fostered environments that allowed their children to approach challenges with greater resilience. These kinds of environments—characterized by consistent love, understanding, and realistic expectations— made their children more confident about facing life's challenges.

Creating an Emotional Safe Haven

For children with DMDD, a supportive environment is one where they feel safe to express their emotions without fear of judgment or punishment. The Brown family worked hard to create this emotional haven for Liam, establishing family routines that prioritized emotional check-ins where each family member could share their feelings. These moments allowed Liam to express his emotions in a controlled, supportive environment where he could feel more secure and understood.

The Gupta family also focused on creating an emotional haven for Anika by encouraging open conversations about feelings. They clarified that no emotion was "wrong" or "bad," helping Anika feel comfortable expressing her feelings without fear of a negative response. This open communication reinforced a sense of trust between Anika and her parents and made her feel more supported and understood.

Encouraging Open Communication

Open communication is critical to building a supportive environment. The Morgan family made it a priority to encourage Maya to talk about her feelings, even on days when things didn't go well. They created a nightly routine where each family member would share one thing they were grateful for and one challenge they had faced that day. Involving the entire family in this practice helped Maya feel heard and valued even when she was struggling with her emotions.

Similarly, the Brown family adopted an open communication policy with Liam—he knew he could come to them with any concerns or emotions he was struggling with. This open door policy helped Liam feel like his feelings were valid and worthy of discussion, reducing the shame and frustration he often felt during his emotional outbursts.

Challenges to Acceptance and How to Overcome Them

Parenting a child with DMDD presents unique challenges that can be overwhelming for families. The emotional volatility, frequent outbursts, and difficulty regulating moods can leave parents feeling helpless, frustrated, and exhausted. However, understanding these challenges and approaching them with the practical strategies we've described in this chapter can significantly and positively impact the child's development and the family's overall well-being. When parents subscribe to the belief that their child with DMDD is not able to control their moods and behaviors at the current moment but—with support—*will* be able to do so in the future, parents are more likely to communicate a sense of acceptance and unconditional love.

Emotional Exhaustion and Burnout

One of the most common challenges for parents of children with DMDD is emotional exhaustion. We discussed this issue in an earlier chapter, but it's worth revisiting. The unpredictable nature of a child's mood swings can lead to constant tension in the household, leaving parents feeling physically and emotionally drained. Parents may feel like they're walking on eggshells, always on alert for the next emotional outburst. This constant state of hypervigilance can be overwhelming, and their feeling of helplessness is likely to grow as they try to manage their child's intense emotional needs.

Parents often start feeling as though their own emotions are being controlled by their dysregulated child. When a child is chronically irritable or has a sudden outburst, it's easy for parents to feel engulfed by this emotional dysregulation and wind up feeling extremely anxious and distressed. It takes an enormous amount of energy for parents to stay calm and not let their child's emotional state consume them. Amid the never-ending advocating for, managing, and attending appointments for their child (with psychiatrists, therapists, professionals versed in various forms of therapy, school staff and officials, etc.), parents often let their own medical appointments go by the wayside due to pure exhaustion and lack of time. Take the case of Sarah and her son Liam—she found herself constantly bracing for his next outburst, which could be triggered by something as small as an unexpected change in plans. The constant emotional strain took a toll on her well-being, leaving her exhausted and unable to recharge.

To cope with situations like Sarah's, parents must prioritize self-care and find ways to recharge and de-stress, even for brief periods. Sarah found relief in scheduling regular breaks where she could unwind, such as taking time to sit with a cup of tea, exercise, read, or even meditate, allowing her body and mind to recuperate from the ongoing demands of parenting a child with DMDD.

Support systems are also invaluable—reaching out to family, friends, or professionals who can help share the emotional burden can prevent burnout. Sarah eventually joined a local parent support group, where she connected with others facing similar challenges. Exchanging coping strategies and shared experiences helped her feel less isolated.

Difficulty with Communication

As we previously noted, children with DMDD often struggle to verbally express their emotions, leading to frustration for both the child and their parents. This lack of communication can intensify the child's emotions and often result in them having outbursts when they feel misunderstood. Parents may find it challenging to de-escalate the situation since they don't know what their child is experiencing internally. This communication breakdown can strain the parentchild relationship, leading to more frequent conflicts and a loss of acceptance.

As an example of this, Raj and Priya struggled to understand why their daughter Anika would suddenly become furious over what seemed to be minor frustrations, like not being able to find her favorite toy. Not surprisingly, Anika couldn't explain what had triggered her anger, so her parents were left feeling confused and unsure about how to help her.

Reflective listening can be an effective technique to address these kinds of communication difficulties. Raj and Priya tried to mirror Anika's emotions, saying, "It seems like you're upset because you can't find your toy." Their acknowledgment of her feelings permitted Anika to feel understood and gradually opened up space for more productive conversations. And again, nonverbal communication is equally important. When words fail, a simple touch on the shoulder or holding a child's hand can provide reassurance and help them feel less isolated in their emotional struggles. Raj and Priya found that sitting quietly with Anika during her emotional storms—without making any attempt to try to fix the problem immediately—often calmed her down faster than any verbal reassurance could have.

Public Meltdowns and Social Stigma

Managing emotional outbursts in public places is one of the more challenging aspects of raising a child with DMDD. Public meltdowns often draw attention, and fear of being judged by others can add another layer of stress for parents. The social stigma associated with these outbursts can make parents feel disparaged or inadequate, exacerbating their already strained emotional state. In some cases, parents may even begin to avoid public outings altogether, leading to social isolation for them and their children.

Michael and Sarah faced a particularly tough experience when their son Liam had an explosive outburst in the middle of a crowded grocery store. Liam was overwhelmed by the store's sensory overload, and when Sarah denied his request for a candy bar, his frustration erupted into a full-blown meltdown. Other shoppers' comments humiliated Sarah, adding to her stress.

Preparation is critical to avoiding or minimizing these public meltdowns. Michael and Sarah started using a visual schedule to help Liam understand what was going to happen during their outings, reducing his anxiety. In addition, providing a five-minute heads-up before any significant transitions were going to happen helped him feel more in control. Despite all their efforts, however, outbursts still occasionally occurred. In those moments, Sarah learned to focus solely on Liam's well-being rather than on the judgment of others. She was able to remain calm and composed—even when faced with public scrutiny—by reminding herself that the goal was to support Liam through his emotional storm.

One mother shared what she did when preparing her son for upcoming events. "From my experience, telling my son what to expect and what not to expect is crucial. I still do this today and he's 16 years old, although emotionally much younger. For example, before going to the supermarket, I would often tell him that we're only going to buy what's on our list. That's difficult for him to hear because he's impulsive and loves to shop. He may say at that point, 'Can we buy more ice cream?' I would say, 'Yes, we can buy more ice cream, so let's add it to the list. However, we are *not* buying candy or other items we don't need.' It's certainly a balancing act. When these kids aren't regulated, parents tend to give in to them to avoid meltdowns and embarrassment. It's hard to say no and so easy to just say yes all the time."

Another parent observed, "I've noticed from the online DMDD support groups that most of these kids—including my son—are very strong-willed and great negotiators. They're super smart! But they're much younger emotionally than their chronological age, so that makes things difficult for parents. However, as kids reach stability, it's important for parents to rein in their parental power. While saying no can result in the child becoming better prepared for a situation, it's also important to say yes sometimes, too."

A father of a child with DMDD shared his story and keen observations about planning their family vacation. "When my son was 10, he told everyone we were going to Legoland in Florida. We had never heard of Legoland. He was watching a YouTube video of a family who had gone there and he knew everything about the location. He was just becoming stable on the Matthews Protocol, so my wife and I agreed that we would go to Legoland. Since Legoland was an hour from Disney, my wife and I thought we could add a few days to visit Disney and stay in the park. Well, that didn't go very well at all. Disney was gigantic compared with Legoland and it was sensory overload for our son. We realized after the fact that our son had only researched Legoland, so he knew exactly what to expect, right down to the hotel room. But he hadn't researched Disney, and it was too overwhelming for him. My point is that when kids know what to expect, they're better prepared."

Another parent commented, "On the days when my daughter was much more irritable, I tried to avoid going to the store or bringing her out in public by myself. I tried to keep a somewhat flexible schedule for store outings—when she was having a particularly good day, I knew I could bring her with less of an issue. That said, sometimes bringing her out is unavoidable."

During an emotionally charged experience, this mother discovered what helped strangers better understand her situation. "My children and I were traveling and got a flat tire, which obviously was not in our plans. Tired and hot, we walked around Walmart while we were waiting for our tire to be changed. My son was riding in the cart and saw something that he liked, and I said no. That immediately triggered a massive meltdown, with screaming, crying, and him slamming the movable part of the cart back and forth, which led to him having a bloody lip. So now I have a child screaming because he's also hurt.

"Onlookers came and peered at me; I could imagine that it looked like I had hit my child in the face. I turned to the people closest to me and said, 'He has special needs, and he's having a moment.' It was like a lightbulb went off in their head—they said 'Ah' and went on their way. After that, whenever my son was having a major outburst in public, I never hesitated to tell people that he had special needs. Culturally, I feel like that term is used more often to describe autism spectrum disorder, and most people understand that ASD can be very difficult. So can my son. It has worked very well—concerned parents have even asked if there was anything they could do to help. But if I hadn't said anything to them, people would have wondered if they needed to call the police."

With regards to grocery store trips, this mother had found a strategy that worked very well with her impulsive son. "Every trip to the grocery store, I told my son that he could pick out *one* treat. Just one! Usually, within a few minutes of entering the store, he would find something that he wanted and would grab it…but then in the next aisle, he would find something else that he wanted even more. I would then ask, 'Which do you want more? Do you want the brownie bites, or do you want the sugar cereal?' He would then choose between the two, and we would move on. Sometimes he would switch out what he had in his hand for another item.

"By the end, there were usually still items I didn't intend on buying in my cart, but he always had just *one* item in hand when we left the store. We started this when he was about three, and I still use this tactic today even though he's almost 14. It allows him to be somewhat impulsive without me having to tell him no. Instead, *he* is making the choices and I don't have to tell him no—I just ask him, 'Which do you want more?' I find ways of telling him no without saying no all the time, and this approach is one workaround."

> A parent in a DMDD support group mentioned that she would never give her son a multi-vitamin with copper in it because she noted increased aggression. When other parents noted the same, I decided to research it myself. I learned that it is common for children with ADHD (which my son has in addition to DMDD) to have low levels of zinc and there was, in fact, a connection with copper. Having low zinc and a higher-than-normal level of copper could create an imbalance of these two minerals, which are associated with dopamine metabolism. One study found that low levels of zinc was linked to higher hyperactivity, anxiety and conduct problems. After having my son's zinc and copper levels checked, results showed both were within the normal range. However, I noticed that his zinc was on the low side of normal, and his copper was on the high side of normal. To balance this out, I give him a zinc supplement (along with B6 and magnesium), since all three are known to possibly help ADHD. I discovered that research conducted by the Walsh Research Institute goes into more detail on this finding.

Let's Return to Barry

Finding the proper treatment for children with DMDD is often a long and complex process. Different medications and therapies may work temporarily, only to lose their effectiveness over time, leaving parents feeling disheartened and unsure of how to proceed. That's what happened to Barry: he was placed on ADHD medication and it worked for a few years, but then as he entered puberty, the effectiveness of the medication waned and his irritability returned. The emotional roller coaster created by inconsistent medication response can make parents and their children lose hope. When this occurs, exhausted, disheartened parents may become increasingly frustrated and angry with their child *and* with themselves, lessening their capacity for expressing unconditional love.

Discovering the proper treatment can feel like an endless cycle of trial and error. Barry's parents were no exception to this—they experienced both relief and frustration as they experimented with different medications. Some provided temporary stability, but their side effects (weight gain, irritability) eventually outweighed the benefits.

Patience and persistence are vital in this process—parents must remain open to the idea that finding the proper treatment takes time and that setbacks are part of the journey. Barry's mother Carol is a strong advocate for her son and spent much time educating herself about DMDD and its treatment protocols. When one treatment stopped working, she sought a second opinion, and after doing more research, she convinced their psychiatrist to place Barry on the Matthews Protocol. That ultimately led to him improving significantly.

Carol shared, "I know deep in my bones that if we hadn't learned about Dr. Matthews Protocol, someone would have been seriously hurt and my son would have been hospitalized—or more likely put in jail. It's been three years since we started the Matthews Protocol, and his rages and constant irritability are just a blur. I can see how his brain is growing and developing as his functionality improves! We have a long way to go with Barry as he has additional diagnoses, but now we have peace in our house. Our son's chance at life still feels like a miracle."

Maintaining Consistency in Routines

Children with DMDD often thrive in structured environments, but maintaining consistent routines can be difficult when emotional outbursts frequently disrupt plans. Still, inconsistent routines can increase a child's anxiety, leading to further emotional dysregulation. On the other hand, an overly rigid approach can sometimes be counterproductive, especially when the child's emotions are particularly volatile.

The Gupta family struggled to maintain a consistent schedule for Anika. They noticed that her mood swings were often triggered when they asked her to transition from one activity to another, especially when doing so involved a task she didn't enjoy. To address this issue, they adopted a more flexible approach to the structure of her days. Instead of expecting Anika to move from playtime to homework without difficulty, they introduced gradual transitions by giving her a five-minute heads-up before each change.

This simple adjustment helped Anika feel more prepared, and she became less resistant to transitioning between activities. On particularly tough emotional days, Raj and Priya allowed yet more flexibility in Anika's schedule, abandoning her established routine altogether. But it was important for them not to abandon the established routine for several days—they only did so when necessary.

Key Takeaways

Parenting a child with DMDD is a journey that hinges on every parent's deep emotional commitment, patience, and resilience. Unconditional love and acceptance form the bedrock of security for children—with unconditional love and acceptance, children can navigate the challenges of emotional regulation, unpredictable behavior, and outbursts. The establishment of a structured yet flexible routine will also help a child feel secure. For instance, parents can have set times for meals and bedtime, but they should be open to adjusting these if a child is having a particularly difficult day.

Setting realistic goals and expectations is likewise essential. Parents should recognize that the progress of a child with DMDD may look different than the progress of children without such a diagnosis. That's to be expected. By celebrating small victories, though, parents can instill a sense of hope and optimism. Setbacks are part of the process, but by focusing on what children *can* achieve, parents help them build confidence and resilience.

It's critical to convey a child that they're accepted for who they are, not just for how they behave or perform. This sense of unconditional love can help buffer the frustration they may feel from the outside world. At times, others—whether peers, teachers, or even extended family— may not fully understand a child's behavior. By educating others about DMDD, parents can foster greater acceptance and reduce misunderstanding, thereby creating a supportive environment for their child.

When children know they're loved no matter what and when they understand that the expectations placed on them are both fair and achievable, they can face the world with a greater sense of confidence and belonging. Even when children with DMDD are confronted with society's demands, a parent's love and acceptance can provide the support that will help them grow, connect with others, and feel a true sense of self-worth.

The power of unconditional love—paired with setting realistic expectations—is transformative for both parents and children coping with the challenges of DMDD. By focusing on consistent emotional support, celebrating strengths, addressing difficulties with compassion, and creating a supportive environment, parents can build a secure foundation for their child's emotional growth. This foundation helps children manage their emotions, and it nurtures a resilient mindset that will serve them throughout their entire lives.

Chapter 7
Nurturing "Islands of Competence"

Zack and Annie's Story

By the time siblings Zack and Annie Kramer were diagnosed with DMDD, the Kramer household had been in constant crisis. Their mother Linda shared, "Our family has no history of trauma, but my father has bipolar disorder, so maybe there's a genetic component. Both of my pregnancies were full-term and healthy. Zack weighed a solid 9 pounds, and two years later, when I had Annie, she was at a good weight of 8 pounds. I breastfed, fed them nutritious foods, all of it." But Linda and her husband Jake noticed early on that their oldest child Zack was fussy at times and had a very difficult time getting to sleep. Annie, on the other hand, had a hard time with separation, which may have just been a phase. Zack showed developmental delays in his gross motor skills but caught up quickly. "Zack couldn't ride a tricycle until the age of four," said Linda. "But then one day, he just hopped on and rode by himself. He was always cognitively advanced, but he did exhibit aggression with other kids in preschool."

By the time Zack was 11, the Kramers had to frequently restrain him because he would attack them or anyone who was in his way when he was raging. The rages could be triggered by something small or big; his eyes would dilate and get so large that he didn't look like himself anymore. "He was very strong during rages," Linda observed. "Half the time, he couldn't remember what he had said and done. There was absolutely no processing with him—he couldn't be reasoned with or make any choices while he was in that state of mind. All we could do was remove his younger sister Annie and try to keep everyone safe until the rage had passed." During one outburst, Jake received a mild concussion while he was attempting to transport Zack to the hospital without an ambulance. Linda recalled that frightening experience: "While Zack was seated in the back seat, he kicked Jake in the back of the head multiple times before they got to the hospital."

At first, Zack's psychiatrist diagnosed him with only ADHD. After many tearful, pleading phone conversations Linda and Jake had with the psychiatrist during which they described the worsening aggression they were experiencing, the doctor finally prescribed aripiprazole. That did curb Zack's aggression quickly. "The problem, however, was that we had to keep increasing the dosage to get the same results, and Zack gained 40 pounds in the process," Linda explained. "The doctor weaned him off the aripiprazole very quickly without adding another medication in its place, and our son was promptly hospitalized for a week. The aggression during the aripiprazole wean was outrageous! I would honestly compare the intensity of it to the intensity of childbirth."

Zack's first hospitalization was at the age of 11. He had three inpatient stays and three outpatient ones. He was inpatient for a total of three weeks; one week was for the aripiprazole wean. Zack was diagnosed with DMDD at age 11 and then with autism at age 13. In the meantime, their daughter Annie was also starting to have mood issues. "The local hospital told us that it was due to trauma from our situation," said Linda. Annie had become increasingly irritable, lost her friends, quit showering, and sometimes exhibited aggression. "For Annie, the rages were more verbal than physical. They were happening more than once a day and were the kind of tantrums that would give you a severe headache!"

Annie was 10 when she was diagnosed with DMDD. Jake recalled, "We were living in trauma and secret horror and felt like those around us didn't understand what we were going through or feel any empathy for us, not to mention we never had any respite. The loneliness of this diagnosis—and the extent to which it made us feel like we were all on our own—had extended from our everyday life to happening even while we were on vacation. There was no relief, no escaping from it."

Later in this chapter, we'll learn more about how the Kramers brought healing to their family.

The concept of "islands of competence" plays a vital role in fostering emotional resilience, particularly in children facing behavioral or emotional challenges such as DMDD. The term refers to areas where a child naturally excels or demonstrates skill, which gives them a sense of accomplishment and pride. When children focus on what they do well, they can build the emotional and psychological strength they need to tackle more challenging areas of life. These islands of competence become a foundation of self-worth—they're crucial for children like Liam, Anika, and Maya. Each child has unique islands of competence, but identifying and nurturing them required a conscious effort from the Browns, Guptas, and Morgans.

Nurturing these strengths isn't just about finding what a child is good at, it's about ensuring that the child feels valued for those strengths, creating an environment where they can thrive, and ensuring that their successes are recognized and celebrated.

Understanding the Origins of "Islands of Competence"

The term "island of competence" was coined by the second author of this book (Bob), who focused on resilience and self-esteem in children. He then expanded upon that concept with the first author (Sam). Together, we have researched and written extensively on helping children and adolescents develop a positive self-image and resilience, especially those with emotional and behavioral challenges. Our work explicitly addresses how children facing difficulties can build resilience and self-esteem despite their struggles.

We (and others) discovered that even children who face significant emotional regulation issues feel competent in certain areas. While these competencies might not align with traditional markers of success, they serve as crucial foundations that allow children to build confidence and resilience. For children with DMDD—who often experience intense emotional storms and feel defined by their negative behaviors—identifying these islands of competence offers a positive counternarrative. Our professional work has revealed that children with emotional dysregulation often internalize their outbursts and frustrations, which unfortunately leads to a pervasive sense of failure or worthlessness.

Recognizing this, we advocate for a strengths-based approach that focuses on nurturing a child's existing competencies no matter how unrelated they may seem to the child's emotional struggles. For instance, a child might excel in art, sports, or solving puzzles. By recognizing these talents, parents and caregivers can help children perceive themselves as being capable and successful in at least one area of their life.

Our approach emphasizes that success in even one area can foster self-esteem and resilience, with positive experiences in one domain potentially leading to growth in others. Parents, caregivers, and educators can create opportunities for children to experience achievements and provide them with moments of pride that reshape their self-perception.

Moreover, we've found that when children are encouraged in their areas of competence, they're more likely to engage in new activities and develop additional skills. For instance, a child praised for their artistic abilities might gain the confidence to explore new interests they had previously avoided.

For children with DMDD, emotional crises can often overshadow their strengths. Still, the concept of islands of competence offers a way for children to focus on their abilities. By nurturing these strengths, parents can help children build the resilience they need to manage emotional challenges and develop a more balanced, positive self-view.

The islands of competence framework represents a transformative shift in perspective. Instead of centering attention solely on areas where a child may struggle, this approach emphasizes the importance of identifying and celebrating small successes no matter how modest they seem. For children with conditions like DMDD, this shift offers a hopeful and optimistic outlook for their future.

Over time, the islands of competence framework can profoundly impact a child's selfconcept and potential. It opens the door to new possibilities for learning, trying new activities, and experiencing success in a variety of domains. As the child begins to feel more capable, they're more likely to take risks, try new things, and build a broader base of competence, reinforcing the cycle of positive growth. The long-term positive impacts underscore the enduring benefits of this approach.

For example, although Liam was prone to emotional meltdowns, he showed an affinity for constructing complex Lego models. This was an early indicator of his problem-solving and engineering-oriented mind, an island of competence that gave him a respite from his frustrations with schoolwork. Once Michael and Sarah acknowledged and encouraged this strength, they began to view Liam in a more balanced light. His outbursts didn't define him—instead, his problem-solving skills and creative thinking became central to his identity.

Similarly, Anika excelled in art. Drawing became her way of processing emotions, a calming mechanism that helped her navigate the intense anger and frustration that so often bubbled to the surface in her interactions with her older brother Arjun. Raj and Priya learned to carve out time for her to pursue this passion, creating a corner of her world where she felt successful and in control.

And then there's Maya. She had a natural gift for nurturing others, especially the family's pets. David and Elena discovered that Maya's irritability and emotional volatility diminished when she was responsible for the well-being of another living creature. Whether she was feeding the family cat or caring for her small garden in the backyard, Maya found peace and emotional comfort in these activities, providing her with an island of competence that helped balance her emotional struggles.

> We could identify something our son excelled at through his tendency to elope when angry. We often had to stop him from climbing onto the house's roof and jumping off. We joined a ninja warrior gym, and he was able to focus his energy and athleticism on climbing and launching into the air, but in a much safer and controlled environment. He made the competitive ninja team and was very proud of himself for every goal he accomplished, like finally getting to the top of the warped wall.

Strategies for Nurturing "Islands of Competence"

Identifying a child's island of competence is only the first step—parents and caregivers must then learn how to foster these strengths in a way that builds resilience and reinforces selfworth. There are several strategies to consider when nurturing islands of competence:

Recognize and Celebrate Small Successes

Acknowledging even the most minor of achievements is essential for children, especially those dealing with emotional regulation challenges like DMDD. These children are often accustomed to receiving criticism or correction because of their frequent emotional outbursts, reactions that lead them to feel like they are constantly in the wrong. Shifting the focus from their struggles to their successes can make a profound difference in how they perceive themselves. Celebrating their accomplishments helps them understand that while they have difficulties, they're also capable of doing things well. This realization can significantly boost their self-esteem and resilience.

Liam's parents made a concerted effort to recognize his talent for following complex Lego instructions. While that might seem like a small or inconsequential skill to some, it was something Liam excelled at. His parents began taking pictures of his completed models. They displayed them around the house, making his Lego creations a visual reminder of his competence. This simple recognition gave Liam a sense of pride and achievement that he hadn't experienced in other areas of his life, such as at school, where he struggled more frequently. The emphasis on celebrating his success with Legos created a positive feedback loop that gradually reduced his feelings of failure and frustration.

Similarly, Maya had a particular affinity for caring for animals, a trait that her parents recognized and celebrated. They observed how much better the family pets seemed to be when Maya took responsibility for their care, frequently reminding her of her competence and commitment. This recognition made Maya feel proud of her abilities and reinforced a positive sense of self-worth. Her parents' consistent praise created a feedback loop, much like in Liam's situation. Maya's pride in her caregiving abilities contributed to fewer emotional outbursts in other areas of her life—as she focused on what she could do well, she felt more in control and less overwhelmed by her emotional struggles.

Recognizing and celebrating small successes isn't just about boosting a child's mood at the moment—it has lasting effects on how they view themselves. When parents, teachers, and caregivers make a point to celebrate these moments, it shifts the child's internal narrative from one focused on failure to one that highlights their strengths. This positive reinforcement helps children like Liam and Maya see that they are indeed capable in certain areas, and that realization can have a ripple effect in other parts of their lives. Over time, these children are more likely to approach challenges with greater self-confidence and resilience because they know they can succeed.

Celebrations of small victories remind children that success isn't always about achieving grand milestones—it's often more about consistently building on small, meaningful moments of competence. Whether completing a Lego set or caring for a pet, these successes form the foundation for a healthier self-image and greater emotional stability, helping children like Liam and Maya navigate the complexities of their emotional lives with greater ease and confidence.

Create Opportunities for Mastery

Children benefit significantly from having regular, predictable opportunities to engage in activities where they feel competent and in control. These experiences are significant for children with emotional regulation challenges because although they often feel like they lack control over their emotions, when they're allowed to excel in specific areas, they develop a sense of mastery related to their skills and abilities. This is crucial for helping them build confidence and resilience! It fosters the feeling that they can in fact influence their environment and outcomes rather than being defined solely by their emotional struggles.

Providing opportunities for mastery is particularly valuable for children like Anika, whose emotions can often feel overwhelming and uncontrollable. When Priya and Raj noticed that she had a natural affinity for artistic expression, they created a dedicated art station in their home. This small space became her sanctuary, where she could retreat whenever she felt emotionally overwhelmed. By giving her the freedom to paint, draw, and create at her own pace, her parents enabled her to channel her emotional energy into something productive and calming. As Anika spent more time at her art station, she honed her skills and began to take pride in her artistic abilities.

The more Anika practiced, the more confident she became about creating something beautiful. This growing mastery over her art allowed her to feel a sense of accomplishment that counterbalanced her frustrations in other areas of her life, like her social interactions and schoolwork. By giving her the space and time to focus on her strengths, her parents helped Anika develop an internal reservoir of positive feelings that she could draw on when faced with emotional challenges. Her art station became more than just a place to draw—it became a safe space where she could experience a sense of control and a feeling of competence, both of which were essential to her emotional well-being.

Similarly, Liam's parents recognized the importance of creating opportunities for him to experience mastery in areas that brought him joy and a sense of accomplishment. Liam had always shown an interest in building things, and his ability to follow complex instructions and build intricate structures gave him a sense of control he didn't often feel in other areas of his life. Understanding the value of this, his parents set aside time each week when Liam could work on new Lego projects without interruption. This became a predictable routine, offering him a structured opportunity to immerse himself in an activity where he felt capable and successful and—notably!—calm.

Michael and Sarah took additional steps to reinforce his feelings of accomplishment. Along with displaying his Lego creations around the house, they also took photos of each finished project and made them into a Lego scrapbook. These displays of his creations highlighted Liam's achievements and provided him with visual reminders of his competence and creativity. By acknowledging and reinforcing his skills in building, his parents were able to nurture his self-esteem, and the sense of mastery he developed through these projects carried over into other areas of his life, helping him approach new challenges with greater confidence.

As Liam continued to engage in his building projects, his parents noticed a reduction in his emotional outbursts. Having regular opportunities to focus on an activity where he felt skilled allowed him to release some of the tension and frustration that had built up in other parts of his life. This sense of mastery provided Liam with a creative outlet and helped him develop greater emotional regulation over time. His Lego projects became more than just a hobby—they became a crucial tool for helping him manage his emotions and build resilience in the face of adversity.

For children with DMDD or similar emotional challenges, these opportunities for mastery—whether through art, building projects, or other activities—serve as a foundation for developing resilience. The more they experience success in one area, the more confident they become in their ability to handle other challenges that come their way.

Set Realistic Expectations and Celebrate Effort

Setting realistic goals is critical for children, especially those who struggle with emotional regulation issues. These children often feel overwhelmed by the pressure of meeting unrealistic expectations, which can lead to frustration, anxiety, and feelings of failure. Unrealistic goals can exacerbate their emotional difficulties, making them feel as though they can never succeed. To counteract this, parents and caregivers must set attainable goals within the child's reach to help them experience success rather than failure. Celebrating effort rather than focusing solely on an outcome is a powerful way to reinforce the idea that persistence and dedication are valuable even if the results are imperfect.

For children with emotional regulation challenges, it's essential to acknowledge that success may not always be immediate or linear. Instead, their development often involves small, incremental steps forward that are punctuated by setbacks and emotional outbursts. By setting realistic expectations, parents can help reduce the pressure these children feel and therefore make their journey toward success more manageable. More importantly, by celebrating their efforts, parents can teach their children that trying and persevering are successes in and of themselves regardless of the outcome. This shift in focus helps children develop resilience and a positive self-image as they begin to understand that their worth is not defined solely by their achievements but also by their effort and dedication.

Maya's parents recognized that setting realistic expectations was vital in helping her build confidence and competence in caring for the family pets. Rather than focusing on perfect behavior or flawless attention to detail, David and Elena praised her consistency and willingness to take on the responsibility of feeding the animals and cleaning their spaces. While Maya's attention to detail was sometimes lacking, her parents didn't criticize her for these minor imperfections or resort to a judgmental statement like "If you tried harder to remember what to do, you could do it, but you're not trying hard enough." Instead, they celebrated her commitment to caring for the pets, reinforcing the idea that realistic effort and persistence are more important than achieving perfection. This approach helped Maya develop a stronger sense of responsibility and pride in her abilities as she learned that competence grows through consistent effort.

Maya's experience also highlights an important lesson for children with emotional regulation challenges: success is not always about getting things right the first time. Instead, it's about showing up and trying even when doing so is difficult. It's about parents and other caregivers *not* assessing a child's level of effort by the end result. Maya's parents helped her understand that mistakes and imperfections are part of the learning process. This perspective allowed her to feel more comfortable in her role as a pet caregiver, reducing her anxiety about making mistakes and encouraging her to continue taking on responsibilities. As a result, Maya became more resilient—she learned that effort is valuable and that improvement comes with time and practice.

Similarly, for Anika, setting realistic expectations was crucial in helping her manage her emotions and feel successful in her creative pursuits. Given her emotional challenges, Anika's parents recognized that expecting her to create perfect art pieces or express herself calmly and in a controlled way wasn't realistic, so instead, they focused on encouraging her to engage with her art consistently. That provided her with a safe space where she could explore her emotions through creativity. Rather than critiquing her work or pushing her to improve quickly, her parents praised her effort and her commitment to her artistic process.

By celebrating Anika's willingness to return to her art station even when she was feeling emotionally overwhelmed, her parents reinforced the concept that engaging in a task *is* a form of success. Anika began to take pride in her ability to manage her emotions through art. This approach helped her feel more in control of her feelings as well as more confident in her abilities as an artist. Like Maya, Anika learned that competence doesn't happen overnight—it grows through consistent effort and dedication.

With Liam, too, his parents took a similar approach to help him manage the pressures he felt in both his academic and personal life. Liam often struggled with emotional outbursts and frustration in school and felt an overwhelming sense of failure when he couldn't meet the high expectations his teachers and peers had set for him. Realizing this, Michael and Sarah shifted their focus from his academic performance to the efforts he made to complete his homework and projects. Rather than expecting perfect grades or flawless assignments, they celebrated Liam's dedication to attempting to do the work even when it was difficult.

When Liam was assigned a challenging science project, his parents didn't emphasize the need for him to execute it perfectly or receive top marks. Instead, they focused on his efforts to research the topic, gather materials, and complete the project regardless of the outcome. They praised his perseverance and problem-solving skills, reminding him that working through challenges is as important as achieving high marks. This encouragement helped reduce Liam's anxiety about future projects and allowed him to approach challenges with a greater sense of calm and determination. When he received a passing grade rather than top marks, his parents still celebrated his hard work, once again reinforcing the value of effort over perfection.

Through this approach, Liam internalized that trying and persisting even when tasks are complex is a form of success. This shift in mindset helped him manage his frustration and reduce the frequency of his emotional outbursts, as he no longer felt the pressure to be perfect. Slowly, Liam became more confident in tackling complex tasks, knowing that his effort would consistently be recognized and celebrated even if the results were imperfect.

In all three examples—Maya, Anika, and Liam—the parents' focus on setting realistic expectations and celebrating efforts rather than outcomes noticeably impacted their children's emotional well-being and sense of competence. By hearing their parents acknowledge that success is not always about perfection but *is* about persistence and effort, these children were able to build resilience and confidence in their abilities. This approach not only reduced their anxiety and frustration but also helped them develop a more balanced and positive self-image.

Encourage Social Reinforcement

> We started noticing that our son had a special way with animals. Every shop owner who brought their dog to their business knew our son. Our son would stop in for a few minutes to greet their pet and soon began conversing with the owner. Animals met his emotional needs and were a way to connect with others. With each visit, our son's confidence grew, and so did his socialization skills. On weekends, we look for opportunities to build on this strength. Our family outings have included spending time on an alpaca farm, visiting with baby piglets, therapy horse lessons, and walks and yoga with therapy dogs. It's been amazing to witness animals' healing power on our son and how they have helped him grow in many areas.

Social reinforcement is a powerful tool in building a child's confidence and self-worth, especially for children who face emotional or behavioral challenges. When other people— teachers, friends, extended family—recognize and validate a child's competence, it adds crucial layers to their developing sense of self. While praise from immediate family members is essential, when people outside the family also acknowledge a child's abilities, that can provide external validation that reinforces the child's strengths. This external recognition signals to the child that their competence is visible and appreciated within a broader social context. This recognition can be incredibly affirming.

Social reinforcement offers a form of validation that can extend beyond what parents provide at home. When children hear positive feedback or acknowledgment from someone like a teacher or family friend, they're likely to begin to internalize the message that their skills and efforts are not just valued within the family but also by the larger community. This kind of reinforcement can be particularly impactful for children who feel isolated in their struggles— such recognition shows them that their strengths are meaningful to others.

In Anika's case, her art teacher became a critical part of her support system at school. From early on, the teacher recognized Anika's artistic talent and wanted to highlight her abilities in a way that went beyond verbal praise. When the teacher displayed Anika's artwork in the school hallway, for example, that gave Anika a moment of recognition that extended beyond the classroom. This act of social reinforcement was a mighty one for Anika, as it showed her that her talent was worth sharing with the entire school community.

The display of Anika's artwork became a point of pride for her and her family. When her parents visited the school to see her artwork on display, their actions further reinforced the message that Anika's talents were valued by others outside of the family. This shared experience of public validation strengthened her sense of competence and self-worth—Anika could see that her skills and efforts were acknowledged by others. That encouraged her to continue pursuing her art. Receiving social reinforcement from her teacher as well as her parents helped Anika build a stronger identity as an artist, boosting her emotional resilience.

Liam also benefited greatly from social reinforcement, mainly through family and friends who recognized his unique abilities with Legos. His parents had long supported his passion for creating intricate Lego structures, but when friends and extended family began to notice and praise his creations, their appreciation provided a new level of validation for him. For example, family friends frequently invited Liam and his parents over for casual dinners, and during these visits, they asked Liam to show them photos of his latest Lego projects. They would then marvel at the complexity and creativity of his designs. Their genuine praise and interest significantly impacted Liam, greatly boosting his confidence in his skills. The attention and validation from family and friends also allowed Liam to talk about his work and explain his thoughts behind each creation, further reinforcing his sense of competence.

For children like Anika and Liam, social reinforcement is integral in helping them build confidence, resilience, and islands of competence. When teachers, family friends, or other community members acknowledge and validate their talents, it conveys a message that their strengths are valuable and worthy of recognition. This kind of reinforcement is essential in helping children internalize the idea that they are capable individuals regardless of their emotional or behavioral challenges.

Furthermore, social reinforcement encourages children to continue pursuing their passions and skills. Children who perceive that a wider audience appreciates their efforts are more likely to take pride in their abilities and feel motivated to keep improving.

Model Emotional Resilience Through "Islands of Competence"

Parents play a crucial role in helping their children develop emotional resilience, and one of the most effective ways to do this is to model resilience themselves. By openly sharing their own experiences with failure, persistence, and the ability to bounce back after setbacks, parents demonstrate that making mistakes is a normal part of life and that learning and growth are ongoing processes for everyone, even adults. This can be particularly powerful when combined with the idea of islands of competence. When parents discuss and highlight their areas of competence—skills or talents they've developed through effort and persistence—they show children that success is not about perfection but continually building on strengths.

Children with emotional regulation challenges often struggle with feelings of inadequacy because they face frequent emotional storms that leave them feeling out of control. Learning about their parents' islands of competence and how they coped with challenges can be incredibly reassuring for these children. It sends the message that everyone has strengths they can rely on during difficult times and that resilience is not about avoiding failure but about recognizing and building on one's strengths to overcome obstacles.

Elena and David consciously tried to model emotional resilience for Maya by sharing their personal experiences with challenges at work or in other areas of life. They went beyond simply talking about their mistakes or failures—they made it a point to emphasize how they had relied on their own islands of competence to overcome these challenges. When Elena faced difficulties at work, she would talk to Maya about how she had leaned on her organizational skills or her ability to communicate effectively with colleagues to resolve problems. Similarly, David shared stories of how his patience and persistence had helped him overcome project setbacks.

By highlighting these strengths, Elena and David showed Maya that everyone has areas of competence they can rely on when things get tough. This was especially reassuring for Maya, who often felt overwhelmed by her emotional outbursts and struggles in school. Listening to her parents talk about their strengths and how they used them to manage difficult situations gave her a new perspective, and she began to understand that resilience involved identifying and using her own strengths to meet challenges at home and in school. David explained to Maya that when he had a challenging project at work, he used his ability to break down tasks into smaller, manageable steps—his own island of competence—to make the project less overwhelming. He didn't try to hide his frustrations but instead showed Maya how he dealt with them by relying on the strengths he had developed over time.

Maya began to internalize these lessons and apply them to her own challenges. When she faced difficulties at school, mainly in subjects she found frustrating, Maya approached them with more patience and self-compassion. Instead of giving up in frustration, she began recognizing her islands of competence. One of those was being particularly good at organizing her schoolwork and keeping track of assignments. While she may not have excelled in every subject, her organizational skills helped her manage her workload. Realizing that gave her the confidence to tackle more complex tasks. In other words, Maya learned that competence in one area could help her develop in others.

With their new approach, whenever Maya had an emotional outburst at home or struggled with a difficult homework assignment, her parents reminded her of her islands of competence. "You're good at keeping your room organized," they would say. "How can we use that skill to help you with this?" By reframing her challenges within the greater scope of her strengths, Maya felt more empowered and less overwhelmed.

In another example, David shared with Maya how he had struggled with a particular skill at work but had relied on his ability to communicate effectively with his team—a skill he had developed over many years. He explained to Maya that even though he wasn't perfect at everything, he could still contribute to the success of his projects by focusing on his communication strengths. That story resonated with Maya as she began to see that resilience wasn't about excelling in every area but about recognizing and relying on her unique abilities to get through difficult situations.

Challenges in "Nurturing Islands of Competence"

While nurturing islands of competence can powerfully impact a child's development, it also presents a unique set of family challenges. It involves parents navigating a delicate balancing act as they try to support and encourage their child's strengths while managing their limitations. Maintaining this equilibrium can be especially difficult when families face societal pressures that emphasize traditional markers of success—those typically make it more challenging to appreciate a child's unique abilities. Recognizing these strengths can also be challenging when behavioral issues or developmental concerns overshadow them, leaving parents feeling overwhelmed or unsure about how best to foster their child's potential. Overcoming these hurdles requires patience, understanding, and resilience.

Navigating Behavioral Challenges

When a child frequently experiences emotional outbursts, it can be incredibly challenging for parents to look beyond the immediate chaos and recognize their child's strengths. Amid intense emotions, disruptive behavior, and the frustrations that come with managing a child with emotional regulation difficulties, the positives can quickly be overshadowed by the negatives. Parents may be so focused on managing meltdowns that they lose sight of their child's unique skills, talents, and competencies. The child's behavior becomes the focal point, and moments of competence—no matter how big or small—can be missed or overlooked.

This dynamic often prompts parents to focus disproportionately on what's wrong rather than on what's right, but it's crucial to balance addressing challenging behaviors and nurturing their child's strengths. Children with DMDD often feel defined by their outbursts because that's what garners the most attention from adults. When parents only focus on punitive discipline or correcting behavior, children may internalize that they're "bad" or "difficult" or a disappointment to their parents, which can further contribute to their emotional struggles. Parents must consciously make space for positive reinforcement by recognizing their child's strengths, building up their confidence, and showing them that their behavior, while challenging, does not define their entire identity.

For Michael and Sarah, navigating Liam's frequent meltdowns was an overwhelming and exhausting experience—Liam's emotional storms would often erupt without warning, leaving them scrambling to manage his intense feelings. Like many parents, Michael and Sarah were worried about handling Liam's emotional outbursts. They constantly strategized how to prevent the next meltdown or de-escalate his behavior when it spiraled out of control. In the process, they began to focus almost entirely on Liam's disruptive behaviors and their impact on family life. It was difficult for them to see past the immediate stress and frustration to recognize that Liam also had strengths, skills, and moments of competence.

In their attempts to manage Liam's behavior, Michael and Sarah initially fell into the common trap of seeing Liam's meltdowns as the central issue. His emotional outbursts dominated every family event, interaction, and routine. The chaos created by these outbursts made it difficult for them to appreciate that Liam was not solely defined by moments of emotional dysregulation even though outside of these intense moments, Liam demonstrated a variety of competencies that were worth nurturing. He had a natural talent for building complex Lego structures, a remarkable attention to detail in specific tasks, and a deep curiosity about how things worked. Liam shone in these areas, but the frequent emotional disruptions made it hard for his parents to focus on his positive traits.

Michael and Sarah began to shift their perspective by working with a child psychologist. The psychologist helped them understand that while it was essential to address and discipline inappropriate behavior, nurturing Liam's strengths—his islands of competence—was equally important. Through therapy, they learned strategies for managing Liam's emotional outbursts in a way that didn't overshadow his moments of success. The psychologist emphasized that Liam's challenging behavior was only one part of who he was as a person and that focusing exclusively on that behavior would undermine his self-esteem and reinforce the negative cycle of emotional dysregulation.

Michael and Sarah began to balance their focus by acknowledging and celebrating Liam's strengths alongside addressing his behavioral challenges. Instead of seeing what amounted to punitive discipline as the sole priority, they started looking for opportunities to praise Liam's efforts and talents, particularly in his areas of interest. Whenever Liam completed a problematic building project or demonstrated patience while working on something he loved, his parents pointed it out and celebrated these successes. Over time, this shift in focus helped Liam feel more confident and valued, reducing the frequency and intensity of his meltdowns. He began to see himself not just as a child prone to outbursts but as someone with genuine skills and strengths that others admired.

A critical lesson that Michael and Sarah learned was that discipline doesn't have to be solely punitive—it can also be instructive and balanced with positive reinforcement. By reducing their punitive approach when Liam displayed inappropriate behavior and instead nurturing his strengths, they created a more supportive and encouraging environment for him. When Liam had a meltdown, they addressed the behavior calmly, explaining why it was inappropriate and setting clear boundaries. After de-escalating the situation, they redirected the focus to something Liam had done well recently. Whether they praised his creativity with Lego designs or acknowledged his patience with another activity, this positive reinforcement promoted Liam's internal belief that his strengths were seen and valued.

As Michael and Sarah became more adept at reducing punitive discipline and employing a more positive, nurturing approach, they noticed that Liam's emotional outbursts began to decrease in frequency and intensity. The more they spotlighted Liam's islands of competence, the more confident and emotionally regulated he became. His sense of self-worth grew and he began to take pride in his talents, knowing that his parents saw him as more than just a child prone to meltdowns.

A few years ago, my son had difficulty getting and staying asleep. I read that calcium and magnesium, when taken together, may support staying in the sleep cycle and added to his nightly routine, including a sound machine, cooling eye mask, and humidifier. Over time, we added a weighted blanket and a Hug Sleep pod that swaddles and cocoons. Even though we kept a consistent sleep schedule, eventually, 5 mg of melatonin was needed. Last year, I noticed my son's snoring got worse, and he would sit up multiple times throughout the night and told his pediatrician. I learned that poor sleep can have an impact on mood, including anger, irritability, frustration, mood swings, and lack of motivation — and my son was dealing with all these issues. We were referred to a pulmonologist who suspected my son had sleep apnea and ordered a sleep study. The results showed severe sleep apnea, and we were referred to an ENT surgeon. After my teenage son recovered from his tonsillectomy and adenoidectomy, his sleeping improved dramatically. Opening up his airway, improved his breathing and quality of sleep, as well as helping him with better cognitive function and behavior. Research suggests a strong connection between improved sleep quality after surgery and a decrease in the severity of ADHD symptoms. Several months after my son's surgery, his ferritin—a protein needed to store iron in the blood—increased to an optimal level. That was an added bonus since low iron levels can be associated with anxiety, depression, and sleep disorders. Removing his tonsils and adenoids possibly leads to better iron absorption and utilization in the body.

Balancing Competence with Academic Expectations: The Role of Islands of Competence

Balancing a child's strengths with academic or social expectations is a common challenge for parents, especially when their child's natural talents lie outside of traditional academic subjects. This balancing act can be particularly difficult for families who place a high value on academic achievement, as there may be pressure to prioritize school performance over other areas where the child naturally excels. This was the case for Raj and Priya, whose extended family emphasized academic success as a marker of personal worth and future potential. In their family, high grades in math and reading were seen as the path to success—anything less was often viewed as failing.

Anika was highly skilled in art, a talent that brought her joy, fulfillment, and confidence, but her math and reading struggles became a concern, especially in a family that viewed academic achievement as paramount. The pressure on Anika to improve academically began to overshadow her strengths in art, creating a tension between nurturing her competence and meeting family expectations. Raj and Priya were caught in a difficult position—they wanted to support their daughter's unique talents while ensuring that she met the academic standards her family and society had set for her.

It wasn't long before the Guptas recognized that focusing solely on Anika's academic weaknesses would likely damage her self-esteem and undermine her sense of competence. They understood that a child who feels constantly criticized or pressured in areas where they struggle can develop a negative self-image, a perception that may lead to increased frustration, anxiety, or disengagement from school altogether. Thus, Raj and Priya needed to balance supporting Anika's academic development and nurturing the areas where she excelled. For Anika, art wasn't just a hobby, it was a vital area where she felt capable and confident and could express herself and experience success. Raj and Priya knew that fostering this sense of competence was essential for Anika's overall emotional well-being.

To address Anika's academic struggles without diminishing her confidence, Raj and Priya decided to work closely with her school. They sat down with her teachers and discussed how best to support Anika in math and reading while protecting her time for artistic pursuits. The goal was to help Anika improve in the subjects she found challenging without letting those struggles define her self-worth or overshadow her strengths.

Together with the school, Raj and Priya created a plan that included morning tutoring sessions specifically targeted at improving Anika's math skills as well as plenty of time in the afternoon for her creative activities. That way, she could focus on improving her math skills without feeling overwhelmed or deprived of the time she needed to engage in something she loved. This balance was crucial in helping Anika maintain a positive self-image, allowing her to see herself as more than just a student struggling in math—she began to view herself as someone with strengths, an image that ultimately bolstered her resilience in the face of academic challenges.

Anika's parents understood that by emphasizing her strengths in art, they were helping her build a foundation of confidence that would support her in tackling other challenges.

Raj and Priya also worked to involve their extended family in celebrating Anika's artistic achievements—they organized family events where her artwork was displayed, inviting relatives to admire and appreciate her creations. This deliberate effort shifted the focus from sheer academic achievement to a broader recognition of Anika's strengths. Doing so helped alleviate some of the pressure Anika felt and allowed her to feel more valued for her unique talents. Balancing a child's strengths with academic expectations requires a thoughtful approach that nurtures both their areas of competence *and* their challenges. For Raj and Priya, this balancing act meant working closely with Anika's school to provide academic support while ensuring that her struggles in math didn't overshadow her artistic talents. This helped Anika develop the confidence and resilience she needed to thrive in all areas of her life, proving that success isn't defined solely by academic achievement but by a holistic recognition of a child's strengths and abilities.

Focusing Too Much on Competence: The Balance Between Nurturing Strengths and Encouraging Growth

Islands of competence, as essential as they are for the emotional and psychological development of children like Maya, Anika, and Liam, must be carefully balanced with the need to foster growth in areas where the child may struggle. Parents play a critical role in this balancing act—they must ensure that while they nurture their child's strengths, they don't unintentionally neglect the areas where the child needs to develop. While islands of competence offer a foundation of confidence, security, and self-worth, focusing exclusively on them can create blind spots in a child's development. Children must be challenged to step outside their comfort zones and develop new skills in order to thrive holistically.

Islands of competence should serve as a launching pad for broader growth, not as a shelter that prevents a child from addressing their weaknesses. For example, Maya excelled at nurturing family pets and displayed a natural talent for caregiving and responsibility. This is undoubtedly a valuable competence, but if her parents had focused solely on this strength, they might have missed opportunities to help her develop other essential skills, such as improving her social interactions with peers. The challenge for parents is to strike a balance: provide the child with enough support in their areas of competence to boost their confidence and self-esteem while gently encouraging them to work on areas where growth is needed.

David and Elena understood the importance of this balance for Maya. While they encouraged her love for animals and praised her for her consistent efforts in feeding, grooming, and ensuring their pets' well-being, they also recognized that she struggled when it came to her interpersonal skills with her classmates—she found social interactions challenging and often withdrew in social settings, feeling unsure of herself when making friends or participating in group activities at school. While it would have been easy to focus solely on Maya's competence with animals, her parents knew that doing so might reinforce her tendency to retreat into her comfort zone. Competence in one area should not become a shield against developing other critical skills, they realized, so they sought to leverage Maya's strength in caring for animals as a bridge to help her grow socially. They did this by creating low-pressure opportunities for Maya to interact with her classmates, using her love of animals as a common ground to build connections. For example, they invited her classmates over for playdates and gave Maya an opportunity to show them her garden and introduce them to the pets she loved.

These playdates were a success because they allowed Maya to engage with her peers in a comfortable, familiar environment and take pride in her competence while practicing social interactions. Maya's confidence in caring for animals helped ease her anxiety about socializing. Gradually, as she shared her knowledge about pets, she felt more comfortable conversing with her classmates. The social pressure was reduced because Maya was in her element and speaking about something she was passionate about. This approach enabled her to slowly develop her social skills while still drawing strength from her island of competence.

In fostering Maya's interpersonal growth, David and Elena demonstrated a vital parenting principle: nurturing a child's islands of competence must be paired with efforts to encourage development in their weak areas. This ensures that the child will grow holistically and not become overly dependent on their strengths. Overreliance on competence in one area can sometimes be a barrier to growth in other places, leading to uneven development where children avoid situations that expose their vulnerabilities. Maya's parents used her love of animals not as an escape from her social challenges but as a tool to help her overcome them.

Likewise, Raj and Priya were careful not to let Anika's competence in art become a shield that prevented her from improving in school. They recognized that fostering growth in areas where Anika struggled was just as important as celebrating her artistic success, which was why they ensured that parts of her afternoons were still reserved for creative activities even as they enrolled her in math tutoring sessions.

Michael and Sarah encountered a similar situation with their son. Liam's competence in building intricate Lego structures was a source of pride for the whole family. It gave him a sense of control, mastery, and accomplishment, all the more so because his emotional outbursts often made him feel *not* in control in other aspects of life. However, his parents were mindful not to let Liam retreat into his Lego-building world at the expense of developing other life skills. They recognized that while it was important for Liam to have his island of competence to boost his self-esteem, he also needed to work on managing his emotions and building social skills.

To help Liam grow beyond his island of competence, Michael and Sarah gently encouraged him to apply the patience and attention to detail he demonstrated in his Lego projects to other areas of his life. For instance, they used his love of building to introduce him to teambased activities, such as joining a robotics club where he could work with others on engineering challenges. This allowed Liam to continue developing his competence and simultaneously build teamwork and social skills, areas where he needed growth. By expanding the contexts where Liam was able to apply his strengths, his parents helped him grow beyond his comfort zone while leveraging his sense of competence.

Returning to Zack and Annie's Story

When Linda and Jake Kramer came across the Matthews Protocol for DMDD, they were skeptical, but they also knew they had nothing to lose—they couldn't continue living in chaos. "People kept talking online about having great success with this method, so I gathered the documentation and presented it to our physician," said Linda. "She told us not to 'get our hopes up' but said that she would be willing to try it since nothing else had helped Zack. After just a month or two, we saw that the oxcarbazepine was improving his mood, and adding amantadine sharply curbed impulsivity and aggression. It was like a miracle!"

Although finally stable, Zack—who had a history of chronic migraines—started to develop migraines related to the oxcarbazepine increases and had to switch to one of the alternatives with a lower likelihood of causing headaches, lacosamide (Vimpat®). "Our local children's hospital had never used lacosamide in psychiatry, but luckily, our doctor was willing to consult with the neurology department at the hospital and consequently felt more confident trying it," Linda explained. "And it worked! Lacosamide along with guanfacine ER [in this case, an alternative to amantadine in the protocol] are keeping our son stable."

At the same time that 13-year-old Zack stabilized, his 10-year-old sister Annie was rapidly regressing and exhibiting similar behaviors. She too would be diagnosed with DMDD and later treated with the same protocol as her brother, and a short four months later, she too was stable. "Annie does great on the oxcarbazepine and amantadine combo—she only initially experienced temporary side effect issues," Linda reported. "The school called and commented that they couldn't believe the changes they had witnessed! For our daughter, making sure she's at the target serum level of oxcarbazepine has been important for her stability. We make little tweaks and adjustments as needed. We also have guanfacine ER on board for ADHD and escitalopram (Lexapro®) for anxiety." Once Annie's mood was stabilized, a stimulant was added to help her better focus at school. Fortunately, Annie was able to tolerate the stimulant. (Some children with DMDD cannot, even after they have achieved stability.)

Linda and Jake found that once their children had achieved stability, they were better able to notice their strengths. Zack, now 18, graduated from high school last year. His mom observed, "We have occasional bad days, I think largely because of the autism and anxiety, but he's stable. Zack is still somewhat impulsive, but he's not angry anymore. He showers every day and keeps his room clean." Zack held a job for several months at a fast-food restaurant and is now applying to a restaurant chain where he hopes to be employed.

Linda observed, "Zack has a strong interest in archeology and reads everything he can on that topic. Through his enjoyment of books, he's learned a great deal about Egypt, expeditions, and history. We encouraged his interests since he hopes to attend college in two years to earn a degree in anthropology." For years, Zack has also had an interest in music—he played cello in an advanced orchestra and composed songs and is currently taking voice lessons. These days, Zack is composing folk metal, a genre that combines traditional folk music with heavy metal. "My wife and I recently performed one of Zack's compositions with our band, which was a thrill. The feedback was amazing!" said Jake.

Annie, now 15, has her own interests that her parents continue to strongly support. For almost three years, Annie has volunteered at the local library and continues to attend Girl Scouts. At school, she's in honors English and enjoys fashion design and sewing classes. "We noticed how much Annie enjoyed art and created a designated area at home where she can design jewelry, paint, draw, and crochet, which she taught herself," Jake proudly said. Linda agreed, adding, "Annie is artistic, hygienic, and social."

Through the years, Linda and Jake have looked for various art camps for Annie to attend to encourage and develop her natural artistic talents. Linda added, "Annie also enjoys writing anime-related fiction and is part of an online community that has encouraged her work." While both children are doing well and learning life lessons along the way, Linda noted, "We continue to keep up a structure every day since both children require the consistency of routine. That has certainly contributed to their individual successes!"

Key Takeaways

Nurturing islands of competence is important for children with DMDD. Because these children often experience intense emotions and frequent outbursts that make it difficult to feel successful in everyday activities, helping them identify and focus on areas where they excel isn't just about creating moments of success—it's about using those successes to build the emotional resilience they need to navigate the unique challenges of DMDD.

Parents provide a crucial lifeline to emotional regulation for children with DMDD by focusing on their strengths and reinforcing their islands of competence. These positive experiences counterbalance the overwhelming frustrations or failures these children often face. When they're encouraged and given opportunities to develop their strengths, they gain a sense of control and competence, which helps build their emotional resilience and makes it easier for them to cope with the mood swings and emotional outbursts associated with DMDD.

Children with DMDD who experience success in one area begin to see themselves as more capable even in moments when their emotions seem unmanageable. This shift in perception helps foster a growth mindset, where they can believe that persistence and effort will allow them to overcome obstacles. These successes offer more than just temporary boosts in confidence— they act as anchors that children can rely on when they face emotional or behavioral challenges.

Caregivers, parents, and educators play a vital role in celebrating these victories. By recognizing these moments, they help children with DMDD see that they are not defined by their disorder but by their strengths. Over time, these islands of competence grow, allowing children to expand their emotional resilience and better manage the ups and downs of DMDD. This approach equips them with the tools they need to face adversity with confidence and to adapt to changing circumstances.

Chapter 8
Helping Children with DMDD Learn from, Rather Than Feel Defeated by Mistakes

Kellan's Story

Kellan Anderson showed early signs of irritability—it was difficult to soothe him when he was a baby. As he grew older, his irritability worsened, and on top of that, he exhibited extreme sensitivity to clothing, sounds, and other sensory stimuli. Kellan's mom Mindy said, "By the time Kellan was 18 months old, his daycare provider expressed concerns about his behavior, suggesting that he might have ADHD due to his frequent meltdowns and inability to nap." These concerns were particularly alarming to Mindy, who had grown up with a violent brother diagnosed with ADHD and aggression as well as a father with bipolar disorder. Fearing her son might face similar challenges, Mindy became increasingly worried about his future.

Kellan's behavior continued to escalate—he had frequent violent rages, particularly when he was overstimulated or told no. At such times, he significantly damaged classrooms at school and had a history of darting out of the school building, even in kindergarten. On multiple occasions, this led to the police getting involved. At home, his rages were equally severe, leading to fears for his safety and the safety of others. The situation became so dire that Kellan was hospitalized in a pediatric psychiatric ward at the age of five. When he was discharged, Mindy was told to contact them when Kellan needed to return to the hospital, implying that his issues would likely persist. Despite all of this, however, one of Kellan's favorite activities was creating all forms of art, from assembling collages to working with clay. When he was engaged in creating art, his emotional tolerance often seemed to be better.

Even with the grim predictions from the hospital staff, Kellan's mother refused to give up. She then learned about the Matthews Protocol and sought out a doctor willing to try it. But although the anti-epileptic medications and amantadine offered a new approach to treating Kellan's explosive behavior, Kellan's father Anthony was much more skeptical. "Why, after multiple failed attempts at treatment, would this time be any different?" he asked.

Mistakes are an inevitable part of learning. Every child makes them (and every adult, too). Ideally, mistakes become valuable lessons on the path to maturity. However, for children with DMDD, mistakes can often feel overwhelming, triggering intense emotional reactions that seem disproportionate to the error. Rather than learning from these experiences, children with DMDD may feel crushed and spiral into frustration, anger, or despair. For example, Liam struggled with math, and when he made a mistake on a test, he didn't just feel disappointment, it was as if the mistake had confirmed all his worst fears about himself: that he was "stupid" and "incapable." The intense self-criticism that followed quickly turned into anger, which he directed at his teacher and classmates, leading to a breakdown in the classroom. While his peers were able to shake off small mistakes and view them as part of the learning process, Liam's emotional reaction to mistakes felt insurmountable. Without a proper strategy for handling these feelings, each mistake became an emotional catastrophe, not a learning opportunity.

Similarly, Anika often experienced extreme frustration when she couldn't immediately master a new skill, whether that was riding her bike or completing an art project. One afternoon, while attempting to draw a simple picture for a school assignment, she made a mistake with her drawing. Instead of calmly erasing it and trying again, Anika ripped the paper apart and threw her pencils across the room, overcome by rage. In her mind, the mistake wasn't something she could fix, it was an unbearable sign of failure. Like many children with DMDD, her emotional dysregulation made it nearly impossible to focus on solutions when faced with frustration. Even more concerning was that Anika was learning that mistakes were bad and to be avoided at all costs.

Maya faced a similar struggle. While working on a group project at school, she accidentally skipped an important part of the instructions, leading the project to go off track. When her classmates pointed out the mistake, Maya's response was extreme: she immediately felt overwhelmed and spiraled into a state of hopelessness and self-blame. Instead of collaborating with her group to fix the problem, she shut down emotionally, leaving her peers to continue without her. For Maya, the mistake didn't just feel like a small setback—it felt like a confirmation that she would never succeed, further fueling her avoidance of group projects in the future.

These examples illustrate how children with DMDD often experience mistakes differently from their peers. Their emotional responses can be so intense that they become stuck, unable to process the situation rationally. This emotional dysregulation can prevent them from learning valuable lessons from mistakes, which in turn leads to a cycle of avoidance and despair.

> Dyslexia prevents my son from keeping up with his peers when taking notes and participating fully in group projects. Most of the time, it is easier for him not even to try to complete an assignment rather than attempt it and fail. He knows he doesn't put in 100% effort in class and appears unmotivated, but this seems to be easier for him than facing all the feelings of incompetence, failure, and frustration that come with trying to keep up with his peers. He inevitably fails to complete classwork every day, even if he tries his hardest. His perception is it's easier not to try in the first place.

This chapter explores the power of cultivating a growth mindset and how parents can help their children embrace mistakes as part of the learning process. In our research and interactions with families of children who have DMDD, both of us have incorporated fostering a growth mindset as a major component of a resilient mindset. For children like Liam, Anika, and Maya, developing a growth mindset involves reframing mistakes as being opportunities for growth rather than indicators of failure. By fostering perseverance and resilience, parents can transform how their children experience challenges and offer them a sense of hope and control over their emotional responses.

Liam's parents helped him by focusing on his effort rather than the outcome, encouraging him to see that making a mistake in math doesn't mean he's "bad at math"—it means he's learning. With time and support, Liam started approaching math more confidently, knowing that mistakes are part of the process. Anika's parents worked with her to develop strategies to cope with frustration, teaching her how to take a break and return to her drawing after calming down. In Maya's case, her parents and teachers modeled problem-solving behaviors, showing her that mistakes are not the end point but rather a chance to attempt something again.

Without this growth mindset, children with DMDD are likely to continue to struggle with emotional dysregulation and become more prone to avoiding challenges, something that will lead to a lack of personal growth and development. However, with the right support, these children can learn to manage their emotional reactions and view mistakes as a normal and important part of learning. By doing so, they can unlock their potential for growth, resilience, and emotional well-being.

The Growth Mindset: A Path to Resilience

The concept of a growth mindset was pioneered by psychologist Carol Dweck. It has farreaching implications, particularly for individuals facing emotional and behavioral challenges. Dweck's research highlights the difference between a growth mindset and a fixed mindset—two contrasting approaches to personal abilities. A growth mindset is a belief that intelligence and abilities can be developed through effort, learning, and perseverance, whereas a fixed mindset views these traits as static and unchangeable. Individuals with a fixed mindset often feel limited—they tend to interpret failures as manifestations of inherent inadequacy, a perception that can hinder personal development.

In contrast, those who adopt a growth mindset see challenges and setbacks as opportunities for learning and improvement. Research has shown that this perspective fosters emotional resilience and a proactive approach to problem-solving. Children with emotional regulation difficulties may benefit immensely from cultivating a growth mindset. (Of course, all children can benefit from this kind of positive mindset.) Studies have demonstrated that a growth-oriented attitude can help children with dysregulation difficulties better manage frustration, develop greater self-awareness, and build emotional resilience. This mindset enables them to reframe failures as temporary obstacles rather than insurmountable barriers, promoting long-term personal and academic growth.

Further research in educational psychology supports the idea that teaching children to embrace a growth mindset leads to enhanced motivation, improved learning outcomes, and greater emotional well-being.

Understanding the Impact of DMDD on Mindset

Children diagnosed with DMDD face unique challenges due to their frequent outbursts of anger and irritability and their heightened emotional reactions to situations that most children might find manageable. These emotional fluctuations make it difficult for them to cope with everyday stressors, and they may feel overwhelmed by small setbacks or mistakes. Such experiences can lead them to internalize negative beliefs about themselves, reinforcing a fixed mindset. When children like Liam, Anika, or Maya make a mistake, they may be prone to seeing it not just as a singular event but as a reflection of their overall abilities or worth. This can lead to avoidance of challenges, fear of failure, and a pattern of emotional dysregulation where they perceive themselves as being perennially incapable.

As an example, Liam quickly became disillusioned about his ability to do math when he was unable to solve a problem on his very first attempt. Instead of recognizing the potential to learn from the mistake and improve through practice, Liam viewed the difficulty as proof that he was "bad at math" or "not smart enough." This kind of fixed mindset can produce a cycle of discouragement, reinforcing a child's emotional volatility and reducing their capacity for resilience.

The Role of a Growth Mindset in Emotional Regulation

Adopting a growth mindset isn't just about fostering academic achievement, it's also about emotional growth and resilience. When children begin to believe that their abilities can improve with effort and adult support, they're more likely to approach challenges with curiosity rather than fear. For children with DMDD, this shift in perspective is particularly important—it can reduce their sensitivity to setbacks and help them cope more effectively with emotional triggers. A child who learns to view their emotional outbursts as opportunities for growth (as opposed to evidence of failure) is more likely to engage in self-reflection and seek solutions instead of succumbing to frustration.

Parents can help their children reframe their emotional responses to a challenging situation by emphasizing the progress they're making. Instead of focusing on the fact that their child got upset, a parent can highlight how the child was able to calm down more quickly than before or express their feelings more clearly. This type of positive reinforcement helps the child recognize that their own emotional responses can change and improve with practice, reinforcing a growth mindset.

Encouraging a Growth Mindset in Children with DMDD

Parents and educators play a crucial role in helping children develop a growth mindset, particularly children with DMDD. Fostering this mindset can be highly effective when approached with patience and consistency. Below are strategies to help children with DMDD embrace a growth mindset:

Modeling a Growth Mindset in Everyday Interactions

Children are naturally keen observers of their parent's actions, often picking up on subtle behaviors and attitudes that shape their responses to life's challenges. One of the most powerful lessons that parents can impart is how to navigate mistakes and setbacks with resilience and optimism. When parents model this positive mindset—handling their own errors with patience, understanding, and self-compassion—they offer a living example of how to approach challenges. When a parent spills juice at breakfast and says something as simple as "Oops, I'll clean it up and try to be more careful next time," they communicate that mistakes are not a cause for distress but rather opportunities for growth and improvement.

This message becomes even more essential for children with DMDD, who may find it particularly difficult to cope with intense emotions, especially when things go wrong. For these children, witnessing their parents' calm, measured reactions to mistakes can be incredibly grounding. It shows them that mistakes don't define who they are, and it further teaches children that mistakes aren't something to be feared or ashamed of—they're natural and expected and can be managed without judgment. This approach can gradually help children develop more balanced emotional responses as they become more adept at turning mistakes into valuable learning moments, in the process fostering their resilience and promoting their emotional regulation in the face of adversity.

For example, Maya often got frustrated when she was attempting to build a castle out of blocks. (She wanted to put her dolls in it.) One afternoon, after her tower had collapsed for the third time, she threw a block down. Her mom gently reminded her, "It's okay, Maya. We can take a break. Let's think about how to make it stronger and then try again." Instead of reacting with anger, Maya took a deep breath and began rebuilding, this time using more blocks for the foundation to make the tower more sturdy. Experiences like these helped Maya begin to understand that setbacks are part of learning and creativity, and with her mom's patient guidance, she became more resilient, learning to manage her emotions and persevere through challenges.

Praising Effort Over Outcomes

An essential aspect of fostering a growth mindset is praising effort over results—doing so encourages resilience, adaptability, and continuous learning. For children with DMDD, this reinforcement is especially crucial because it shifts the focus away from fixed outcomes and helps them see the inherent value of the process of learning and growing. The frequent emotional outbursts and irritability that are typical of children with DMDD can be exacerbated by feelings of failure or frustration when success is defined *only* by external achievements like getting good grades or winning competitions. Instead of focusing solely on these types of outcomes, parents can offer praise for effort and persistence, saying things like "I'm proud of how hard you worked studying for your test!" or "I noticed how dedicated you were to finishing that project on time!" This type of feedback helps children understand that improvement comes from dedication and hard work, not just from achieving a specific result.

Anika often felt overwhelmed when working on her homework, especially when she didn't immediately understand the material. After one particularly challenging science assignment, her father noticed that she was getting upset and was ready to give up. Instead of focusing on whether her answers were correct, Raj said, "Anika, I think it's great how long you stuck with this problem and how you kept trying different ways to solve it. That's what really matters!" Hearing this, Anika began to see her effort as an accomplishment in and of itself. Slowly, with consistent encouragement that focused on her perseverance rather than the outcome, Anika's emotional outbursts lessened. She began to approach difficult tasks with more confidence, knowing that effort and persistence were just as important as the final result.

One significant caveat when focusing on a child's effort: when a child doesn't seem to be interested in engaging in a task, parents must avoid saying "If you tried harder, you could do better" or "You could control your behavior if you wanted to." In our practice, as we've been told by many young adults—especially those who faced many challenges—when they were children, they were always upset whenever parents or other adults questioned their lack of effort. One young man said, "I always wondered if there was a test for effort since I was often accused of not trying." A seeming lack of effort is typically a sign that a child doesn't yet have the skills to calm down and successfully manage their emotions and behaviors.

A vivid example of what happens to children when they're accused of not "trying hard enough" involved Rob, a very precocious boy. He learned to ride a bike at the age of three and started reading at the age of four. He was clearly a very intelligent child, but he was also hyperactive and vulnerable to destructive behaviors: he was defiant and aggressive, prone to running away and throwing raging fits when things weren't going his way. His parents, Beth and Roger, were overwhelmed by their son's behavior, especially as they were also raising three other young children. Roger stated, "Rob needed to try harder to behave!" and said that Rob was ignoring parental guidance by not making any effort. Roger assumed that because Rob was a very smart kid, he obviously knew he was behaving badly—he was "choosing" to be mean to his siblings and rageful when he didn't get what he wanted. Roger frequently referred to Rob as his "problem child" and a "wild horse that needed to be broken." The problem was intensified by Roger's perception that his son's behavior was a negative reflection of himself as a parent.

Roger was also disappointed by Rob's lack of effort when it came to many of his activities, from Boy Scouts to sports teams. Roger believed that Rob was a gifted athlete, but what he didn't understand was that Rob frequently would not stick with *anything* just to avoid Roger's criticism. Rob felt like he was never good enough in his father's eyes, so he eventually quit all sports and activities.

Rob had internalized how his dad felt about him very early on. Roger never missed an opportunity to correct Rob, and he made certain that Rob knew how disappointed he was in him. By the time Rob was a teenager, he started owning the label his father had given him. It opened the door to a lot of self-destructive behaviors: drinking and driving, petty theft, being suspended from school. He had very low self-esteem (despite being very intelligent and gifted in many areas) and believed—as did his father—that despite the effort he was putting in, it was never going to be good enough.

Encouraging Realistic Risk-Taking and Learning from Mistakes

Because children with DMDD struggle with intense emotions, they may avoid situations they perceive as being difficult or threatening; this is particularly due to their fear of failure or the potential for emotional outbursts. This kind of avoidance can limit their opportunities for personal growth and learning, and it's why it's so important to encourage these children to embrace challenges within a supportive and understanding environment. When adults like parents and teachers provide encouragement and frame challenges as opportunities rather than threats, children with DMDD are more likely to engage in new activities with a sense of curiosity rather than fear, aiding their emotional and social development.

For instance, if a child is reluctant to participate in a new sport or join a group activity, parents can reinforce the idea that mistakes are a normal and valuable part of learning. By conveying this message, children may gradually become more comfortable with the possibility of not succeeding immediately. This outlook fosters resilience and teaches the child to handle setbacks with less frustration and greater confidence. Over time, these experiences help children with DMDD develop a healthier relationship with challenges, thereby building their emotional flexibility and reducing their fear of failure or emotional outbursts.

Reframing Mistakes as Learning Opportunities

Given that children with DMDD often experience heightened emotional responses to perceived failure—frustration, anger, sadness—teaching them to reframe mistakes can be a powerful tool in helping them manage these intense emotions. For example, when a child struggles with a math problem, a parent can say, "It's okay that this didn't go perfectly today. What's important is that we've learned what didn't work! Now we have a better idea of how to approach it next time."

This approach helps the child focus on the process of learning rather than fixating on the outcome. By emphasizing the value of experimentation and problem-solving, parents can help their children develop a growth mindset, where they view challenges and mistakes as essential parts of learning and improvement. For children with DMDD, this reframing can reduce the feelings of shame and disappointment that often accompany failure and instead build a sense of empowerment and resilience.

Over time, as children internalize this growth perspective, they may become more willing to take on challenges as they will no longer have an overwhelming fear of making mistakes. This shift not only supports their emotional regulation but also encourages a more adaptive, confident approach to learning and personal growth.

Teaching Self-Compassion

Children with DMDD often exhibit harsh self-criticism, which can intensify their emotional distress when they make mistakes or encounter challenges. Teaching them selfcompassion—i.e., treating themselves with the same kindness and understanding they would offer a friend—can be a crucial tool in helping them manage their intense emotions. Selfcompassion allows children to be gentler with themselves, reducing feelings of guilt, frustration, and shame that may follow perceived failures. Over time, this practice fosters emotional resilience and helps children recover more quickly from setbacks.

In the Morgan household, Maya struggled with her growing self-criticism—although she'd once been a bright, joyful child, even small mistakes had begun to trigger intense emotional reactions. One evening, after returning home from school, Maya burst into tears upon realizing she had missed several questions on her spelling test. In frustration, she cried, "I'm so stupid! I can't do anything right!" Elena and David had seen this pattern before and knew they had to intervene. David gently sat beside Maya and encouraged her to take a deep breath, saying, "Maya, it's okay to feel upset, but remember, everyone makes mistakes! You tried your best today, and that's what counts."

This moment was an opportunity for David and Elena to introduce self-compassion to their daughter. Elena added, "Think about how you would speak to a friend if they made a mistake. I'm certain you wouldn't call them stupid. You'd remind them that it's okay, right? So let's talk to ourselves that way, too." Maya hesitated at first but slowly began to internalize her parents' words. They reinforced the concept that making mistakes was a natural part of learning, not a reflection of her worth.

By learning to adopt a kinder, more forgiving perspective, Maya was able to slowly relinquish the intense self-criticism that had plagued her. Over time, practicing self-compassion allowed her to view her mistakes as opportunities for growth rather than reasons to feel bad about herself. This shift helped her to cope more effectively with setbacks; gradually, Maya began to exhibit greater emotional resilience in the face of challenges. Through these compassionate conversations, Elena and David helped Maya develop an inner dialogue that would serve her well as she continued coping with the complexities of DMDD.

Engaging in Reflective Questioning

Rather than immediately correcting a child's mistake, parents can ask reflective questions to shift the focus to problem-solving. For example, when a child is struggling with a math assignment, instead of pointing out what went wrong, parents can ask, "What part of this was most challenging? What can we try differently next time?" This approach encourages children to think critically about the task at hand, fostering a sense of curiosity rather than frustration.

Anika often found math assignments to be particularly stressful. Whenever she encountered a difficult problem, she would quickly get upset, feeling that she wasn't "smart enough" to solve it. Instead of offering a solution right away, her mother began to ask reflective questions such as "What part of this problem are you having trouble understanding?" and "Is there a certain strategy you could use that might help you to solve the problem?" These questions helped Anika approach her assignments with a more analytical mindset; she learned to identify which areas she needed help with and which parts she could figure out on her own.

Depending on a child's age and cognitive level, their parents may need to provide them with some prompts or suggestions to encourage them to consider what they could do differently next time—after all, the default response for many children when asked "What can you do differently next time?" is "I don't know." If that occurs, a parent might say, "Sometimes it's difficult to know what to do differently to correct a mistake. It's something we can try to figure out." Or the parent could respond with, "If you would like me to help out at some point, just let me know." These kinds of questions invite children to reflect on a problem while knowing that adults are available to help them.

Normalizing Mistakes in the Family Culture

To truly cultivate a growth mindset, parents can play a critical role by normalizing mistakes as being part of everyday family life. One effective strategy is to incorporate open conversations about mistakes into daily routines, such as during family meals. At the dinner table, parents can share their own stories of missteps at work or personal challenges they faced during the day and then they can also highlight the valuable lessons they learned as a result. When children hear these kinds of stories from trusted adults, it helps demystify mistakes, showing them that even grown-ups make errors and continue to grow from those experiences.

By modeling this kind of openness, parents communicate that mistakes are not a sign of failure but are an essential part of learning and improvement. This approach also reduces the fear of judgment that children may feel when they make a mistake. In turn, children are more likely to share their own challenges without shame or embarrassment. Encouraging these discussions in a supportive and understanding environment creates a home where mistakes are embraced as opportunities for growth and self-reflection rather than being seen as something to be feared or hidden.

It's important to note that just as parents can serve as positive models for dealing with mistakes, they must be careful not to engage in negative self-talk following a mistake, like saying, "I feel so stupid! I keep making the same mistake over and over again." As we've noted, children are keen observers of *all* of our behaviors, and if they're already struggling with their own feelings of self-worth, our negative self-reflections will only reinforce theirs.

Creating Opportunities for Controlled Risk-Taking

Children who have a deep-seated fear of failure may avoid challenges altogether as a protective measure to prevent disappointment or frustration. This avoidance can hinder their ability to develop resilience and problem-solving skills because they aren't able to practice facing and overcoming difficulties. To counter this, parents can help by providing controlled risk-taking opportunities, situations where mistakes are not only expected but embraced as part of the learning journey. These low-stakes environments allow children to take chances without the fear of harsh consequences, enabling them to learn from their experiences in a safe and supportive context.

For instance, enrolling a child in a creative art class is an excellent way to introduce controlled risk-taking. In such a setting, experimentation is encouraged—after all, there's no right or wrong way to create art. Children can try new techniques, make mistakes, and adjust their approach, all while knowing that the outcome isn't the primary focus. The process of discovery and learning is what matters most. These experiences help children internalize the idea that risk-taking isn't inherently negative and that growth often stems from trial and error.

Why Mistakes Can Feel So Catastrophic

Understanding the emotional landscape that children with DMDD must navigate daily is essential. Emotional dysregulation—a hallmark of DMDD—means that seemingly minor frustrations like a wrong answer in math or a forgotten homework assignment can trigger a flood of emotions. Understanding this reality can bring relief to parents and help them comprehend why mistakes often feel catastrophic. It's not that the mistakes are so severe, it's that the child's emotional response to mistakes is amplified.

For Liam, a simple math problem gone wrong during homework could quickly escalate into a full-blown meltdown. What might have been a minor setback for other children became a signal that he was "bad at math," leading to intense frustration and eventually to him avoiding math altogether. This reaction stemmed not from laziness or willful disobedience but from Liam having a fixed mindset that framed mistakes as evidence of failure rather than an opportunity to learn.

Anika, on the other hand, struggled with social interactions—whenever a friend declined her invitation to play or didn't respond as she'd hoped, Anika felt rejected and unworthy. These minor social missteps felt like personal failures to her. And so instead of learning to navigate friendships with resilience, she began withdrawing from social situations altogether, fearing further rejection. Her fixed mindset made her believe that any social mistake reflected her inability to form meaningful relationships.

Maya's emotional struggles were most apparent in the classroom. If she couldn't immediately grasp a new concept, she would become overwhelmed and tell herself she wasn't smart enough to succeed. This thinking pattern made Maya feel powerless over her learning, leading to frustration and a refusal to engage in tasks that she perceived as being too difficult.

In all three cases, these children saw their mistakes as definitive proof of their limitations. This response is typical of a fixed mindset, where the child believes their abilities are static and unchangeable. In contrast, a growth mindset offers an alternative view: mistakes are not failures but learning opportunities.

Obstacles to Helping Children Learn from Mistakes

Fostering a growth mindset in children with DMDD can indeed be a challenging endeavor. That's because children with DMDD often experience intense emotional reactions and struggle with frustration tolerance, which can make it difficult for them to view mistakes as opportunities for growth. A variety of obstacles contribute to this challenge: a child's natural temperament, the way parents respond to their child's mistakes, societal pressures to succeed, and the child's own internal battles with mood regulation. For example, a child who becomes easily overwhelmed by failure may have difficulty accepting mistakes without feeling discouraged or angry.

Take Maya, for instance. She struggled with frustration whenever she didn't get perfect grades in school. If Maya got a math problem wrong, she often became extremely upset because she believed that she wasn't smart enough. Her parents learned that staying calm and encouraging her to break down the problem into smaller steps helped her see that a mistake wasn't a reflection of her ability but rather a chance to improve.

Anika, on the other hand, found it hard to control her temper when she lost a game during sports practice. When she made a mistake, she often stormed off the field, convinced she wasn't good at soccer. Her parents used a strategy of praising her effort and reminding her that even professional athletes make mistakes. This approach helped Anika slowly start to view her errors as a normal part of learning the game.

Temperament and Emotional Sensitivity

Children with DMDD often have temperaments that make them more sensitive to frustration—because their emotional responses to mistakes can be intense, it's difficult for them to reflect and calmly learn from their errors. Instead, children like Liam, Anika, and Maya are predisposed to react strongly to minor setbacks, which can quickly spiral into emotional meltdowns.

To overcome this obstacle, parents can help their children develop coping strategies to manage their emotional responses before they address the mistake. Liam's parents, for example, began incorporating calming techniques like deep breathing or taking a short break whenever he felt overwhelmed. By learning to regulate his emotions first, Liam was better prepared to return to the task and engage in problem-solving without feeling frustrated.

Parents can also use empathic language to acknowledge their child's feelings without allowing emotions to dominate the situation. Instead of dismissing Liam's frustration, his parents would say, "I know this feels hard right now, but let's take a breath and figure it out together." This approach validated Liam's emotions while creating a space for him to reengage with the problem in a calmer state. His parents also communicated an important message that they were available to help him.

Adverse Parental Reactions to Mistakes

Parents play a crucial role in shaping how their children view mistakes. However, wellintentioned parents can sometimes react in ways that inadvertently reinforce a fixed mindset— conveying harsh criticism, frustration, or impatience can send the message that mistakes are unacceptable, which in turn leads children to fear failure.

In Maya's case, her parents initially struggled with their reactions to her frequent emotional outbursts. When Maya became upset after she'd made a mistake in school, her father sometimes responded with frustration, saying, "You're overreacting! Just calm down and get it right next time." Even though he was trying to motivate her, Maya internalized these comments as pressure to avoid mistakes at all costs, reinforcing her anxiety about failure.

Parents understandably often react to their children's challenging behavior by attempting to manage or correct their outbursts, but this can inadvertently lead to heightened emotional volatility. In response to their children's mistakes, parents mistakenly respond in inconsistent ways—they may react with anger or frustration or use punitive measures like timeouts or punishment in the hopes of quelling disruptive behavior. Although these responses are often well-intentioned, they can escalate the child's emotional state and makes things worse. Children with DMDD have an inherently low threshold for frustration, and punitive or inconsistent responses may only amplify their sense of being misunderstood or rejected.

Additionally, parents may unintentionally model dysregulated emotional responses when they react with frustration themselves. Children with DMDD are highly sensitive to their environment and may mirror the emotional states of their caregivers, thus escalating their dysregulation. Over time, these patterns can create a negative feedback loop where emotional outbursts become more frequent and intense. That's why instead of reacting in punitive or inconsistent ways, it's essential to provide structured, empathic responses that are focused on emotional validation and building skills to better deal with frustration. Without this more nuanced approach, parents risk worsening their child's emotional dysregulation, and that will only serve to reinforce the child's negative behavioral patterns and emotional volatility.

To avoid making the situation worse, Anika's parents introduced the concept of "good enough." They reassured her that things don't always have to be perfect for them to be successful or enjoyable. This helped reduce the pressure Anika felt and allowed her to engage in social situations more confidently. By creating an environment where "good enough" was celebrated, Anika learned that mistakes were not a reflection of her worth but a natural part of building relationships.

Social Comparisons and External Pressure

> My daughter was refusing school, and getting her there was a daily challenge. My goal was to get her to school, no matter when we arrived. One morning, as we drove up to the school, my daughter started to give me a difficult time. I knew only a couple of hours left in the school day. Frustrated, I said the kids had been in class since early this morning. My daughter got angry, shut down, and refused to leave the car. I realized at that moment that she felt like that comparison was highlighting what other kids could easily do (go to school), which magnified what she couldn't do. That day, I learned an important lesson.

Another significant obstacle comes from external pressures, including societal expectations, peer comparisons, or unrealistic standards that the child or their environment sets. When children constantly compare themselves to others, they may feel defeated if they perceive that they aren't performing at the same level. This perception reinforces the idea that mistakes are a sign of inferiority.

Liam, for instance, struggled with feelings of inadequacy when he compared himself to his older sister, who excelled in school. Whenever he saw her succeed effortlessly in areas where he faced difficulty, he felt ashamed of his mistakes and would give up more quickly. This comparison made it difficult for Liam to embrace a growth mindset, as he viewed his mistakes as evidence that he would never measure up.

Parents can help their children overcome this obstacle by fostering a family culture that values individual progress over comparisons to others. Liam's parents began to emphasize that everyone has different strengths and that success looks different for each person. They shared stories about their own struggles and triumphs, too, emphasizing that improvement comes from persistence, not perfection.

By celebrating Liam's achievements and efforts rather than comparing him to his sister, his parents helped him build confidence in his abilities. They also encouraged Liam to focus on his progress rather than worrying about how he measured up to others. This shift in focus helped Liam see that his mistakes were part of his unique learning journey and not a reflection of his self-worth.

> While listening to a psychiatrist being interviewed on a podcast, I learned about the metabolic theory of mental illness, which is the possibility that all mental disorders are metabolic disorders of the brain, based in the mitochondria of neurons and other brain cells. After noticing a positive difference in my son's anxiety after he had been taking magnesium for several weeks, I was curious to know if there was any connection between mitochondria and magnesium. I was happy to learn that magnesium is considered essential in mitochondria (often referred to as the powerhouses of the cell). Without adequate magnesium, the mitochondria cannot efficiently generate energy for the cell

to function properly. Magnesium is required for serotonin production, the "happy hormone" that improves mood, so I give my son 150 mg in the morning and 150 mg at night, along with his medication. Reports indicate that most people are deficient in this mineral due to a poor diet and chronic stress. Magnesium has been shown to help level cortisol—one stress hormone that plays a key role in the body's fight-or-flight response. Since there are many different types of magnesium, selecting the right one or combination is key. Magnesium glycine may help reduce anxiety and improve sleep. Magnesium L-threonate may help with cognitive function and mental clarity, although it can be expensive. Magnesium taurate contains an amino acid called taurine, which has a calming, neuroprotective, and anti-inflammatory effect in the brain. The more I learned about magnesium, I decided to take it as well, to help with my own anxiety and well-being.

Lack of Immediate Solutions

For children with DMDD, the need for immediate gratification or quick success can make it difficult to stick with tasks where mistakes are an inherent part of the learning curve. When children expect immediate results, they may feel frustrated when they don't see instant improvement, a reaction that prompts them to give up rather than persevere through challenges.

Maya often expected that she would be able to do her school assignments quickly, so whenever she encountered difficulties, she would become frustrated and refuse to continue, convinced she couldn't succeed. Her need for quick results prevented her from embracing the long-term process of learning from mistakes.

To address this obstacle, Maya's parents introduced the idea of "process over product." They focused on breaking tasks into smaller, more manageable steps, helping Maya see that progress is gradual and that improvement happens over time. They praised her for sticking with a task even when it was difficult, and they emphasized that learning is a process that requires patience. Instead of focusing on the final grade of a project, David and Elena would highlight how she had improved one specific skill, such as organizing her thoughts or working more carefully.

By shifting the focus from immediate success to gradual progress, Maya learned to appreciate the small victories along the way. That new perspective helped her stay motivated through mistakes.

Back to Kellan's Story

The result of the treatment protocol developed by Dr. Matthews was nothing less than remarkable: within six months of starting the protocol, Kellan's behavior stabilized and the violent meltdowns that had once defined his life ceased entirely.

Kellan could attend school without significant incidents for the first time in years and his family no longer lived in constant fear of his outbursts. Given his history, his psychologist remarked that Kellan was the most "beautifully medicated child" she had ever seen. Kellan has remained stable for seven years and has never had to be readmitted to the psychiatric hospital for irritability and outbursts.

Today, Kellan is 14 and thriving. His behavior is managed effectively, and he leads the life of a typical middle-school boy who plays football and baseball and still loves all forms of art. He is free from the violent rages that once dominated his existence. He is reserved and thoughtful. No one at his current school would ever suspect what he has been through. The protocol has given Kellan a new lease on life, and he looks forward to the future with excitement and optimism.

Looking back, though, Kellan's mother Mindy recognized her son's reluctance to trying new things even when he was in preschool. In order combat this reluctance, Mindy explained, "We would frame these opportunities as a chance to participate in a new sport while being flexible. We said, 'Let's give it a shot for a day and we can talk about it afterwards. If you don't really like it, we can find something else—you don't have to keep going.' This really took the trepidation out of attempting new sports or activities. Kellan's fears had been grounded in the idea that if he tried it the first time and didn't like it, we would keep making him go."

When he was five, Kellan quit soccer mid-season because his cleats and shin guards became unbearable for him due to sensory processing issues. Mindy lamented, "He came to me in the middle of the game, ripped off his cleats, socks, and shin guards, and cried. I didn't force him to continue to play based on the commitment we had made or because I had already paid for the season as I may have done with my non-DMDD child." She accepted the situation and his feelings when he confirmed that he didn't want to play anymore and the reasons behind it. Mindy went on, "Some things can be worked through and other things cannot, such as a sensitivity to the gear required to play the sport. We just decided at that point to look forward to the next opportunity."

Kellan tried many activities along the way, including hip-hop dancing, ice hockey, soccer, baseball, football, a ninja warrior team, and jujitsu. Some activities he decided weren't for him after a single practice; a few he has gone back to after a season. "Flexibility is the key," Mindy said. "Making sure Kellan knew that how he felt about participating would guide what he was involved in helped alleviate his anxiety and helped him be more open to experiencing new things."

The Long-Term Impact of a Growth Mindset

By fostering a growth mindset in children like Liam, Anika, and Maya, parents can equip them with the tools they need to face challenges with resilience. Rather than feeling defeated by mistakes, these children then learn to see setbacks as part of the journey toward success. This shift in perspective reduces their emotional reactivity to mistakes and builds their confidence in their ability to learn and grow.

In the long term, children who develop a growth mindset are more likely to approach challenges with curiosity and perseverance. They understand that their abilities are not fixed but can be developed through effort and learning. For children with DMDD—who often struggle with feelings of inadequacy—this mindset offers hope and empowerment. It gives them the tools they need to handle inevitable setbacks with grace, patience, and resilience.

While many obstacles can hinder a child's ability to learn from mistakes, understanding the barriers faced by children with DMDD is the first step toward helping them overcome their obstacles. By addressing challenges such as temperament, parental reactions, perfectionism, and social comparisons, parents can help their children navigate the difficulties of DMDD with more resilience.

For children like Liam, Anika, and Maya, learning to overcome these kinds of obstacles requires patience, empathy, and a commitment to fostering a growth mindset. Parents can help their children develop the emotional tools they need to persevere through life's challenges by creating a supportive environment where mistakes are accepted and even celebrated.

As Liam, Anika, and Maya's parents learned, mistakes need not be roadblocks—they can be stepping stones instead! Helping children embrace these moments with curiosity and resilience equips them with the outlook they need to navigate the complexities of DMDD and beyond. Mistakes can become part of the learning process and can form essential experiences that build strength, resilience, and hope for the future.

Chapter 9
The Importance of Problem-Solving and Decision-Making Skills for Children with DMDD

Joseph's Story

Joseph Jackson is a 15-year-old boy who struggled with intense mood swings and irritability from a young age. His parents recalled that even as a baby, he had difficulty calming down. His mother Serena shared, "Joseph was highly sensitive to sensory input—loud noises, bright lights, or even a change in his routine could set off inconsolable crying spells. As he grew older, the mood shifts turned into uncontrollable rages that could last for hours." Simple frustrations like losing a game or being told no would result in explosive outbursts during which Joseph would throw objects, scream, and sometimes even hurt himself by punching walls or banging his head against them.

By the time Joseph entered elementary school, his behavior had escalated. Teachers described him as disruptive and emotionally volatile. His grades suffered, and although he was bright and capable, his inability to control his emotions overshadowed his academic potential. His parents sought help from various professionals, initially believing that Joseph had ADHD. He was placed on the stimulant medication methylphenidate (Ritalin®) and then later dextroamphetamine-amphetamine (Adderall®). That helped with his ability to focus but did nothing to ease his mood instability and outbursts.

When Joseph reached middle school, things worsened, as did his fight-or-flight episodes. His puberty exacerbated his emotional swings, and the violent outbursts became more frequent and intense. His parents—feeling overwhelmed and scared for his safety and their own—reached out to a child psychiatrist for a more comprehensive evaluation. After a thorough assessment and review of Joseph's history, he was diagnosed with DMDD.

DMDD was a relatively new diagnosis at the time. "My husband and I felt a sense of both relief and frustration," said Serena. "Relief because they finally had a name for what Joseph was experiencing, frustration because the treatment options were unclear." Joseph's psychiatrist initially prescribed a combination of mood stabilizers and antipsychotics in the hopes of regulating his emotions. While that led to some improvements, Joseph's irritability and rage persisted, leaving his parents in a constant state of anxiety.

After months of trial and error with different medications, Serena stumbled upon an online support group where other parents of children with DMDD shared their stories. Many spoke highly of the Matthews Protocol, saying it had shown remarkable results in stabilizing their children. After discussing the protocol with Joseph's psychiatrist, his parents decided to try it even though their doctor expressed initial hesitation. (DMDD was not yet widely understood in medical circles.)

Joseph's treatment involved a combination of anti-epileptic drugs and amantadine. (The latter is an antiviral medication that's now typically used to treat Parkinson's disease but that has also been found to be effective in managing mood disorders.) Within the first few weeks of starting the protocol, Joseph's parents noticed a significant change. "Joseph's explosive rages diminished in both frequency and intensity," Serena reported. "His mood stabilized and he became more cooperative and less reactive to the everyday frustrations that had previously triggered his outbursts." Joseph himself remarked that he felt calmer and less on edge all the time.

Joseph's improvement was not only noticeable at home but also at school, where he began participating more in class and even made new friends. Joseph's teachers reported a more focused and manageable student, one who no longer disrupted lessons with his uncontrollable emotions. While Joseph still faced challenges, particularly when he needed to manage stress during exams or when things didn't go his way, his progress was undeniable. "Our family no longer lived in constant fear of his next outburst, and our home transformed from a battleground into a more peaceful and supportive environment," observed Serena.

Today, Joseph is thriving. He's working with a counselor to develop coping strategies to handle his frustrations and has even taken up boxing as a way to positively channel his energy. His parents credit the Matthews Protocol for giving them their son back. Joseph's future—once seemingly fraught with crisis—now holds promise and potential. Though Joseph will always need support, he and his family now look forward to a life filled with hope rather than fear.

As Joseph's case illustrates, raising a child with DMDD presents unique challenges. One of the most daunting tasks is teaching children how to make sound decisions and solve problems effectively. For children with DMDD, even small choices and everyday challenges can seem overwhelming, leading to emotional outbursts, impulsivity, and frustration. However, with the proper guidance and structured support, parents can equip their children with the tools they need to approach problems more calmly and thoughtfully.

This chapter will explore a structured framework for teaching problem-solving and decision-making skills to children with DMDD. We'll provide parents with strategies to help their children break down complex situations, consider multiple solutions, and make decisions that reflect thoughtful deliberation rather than impulsive reactions. By developing these skills, children can gain greater control over their lives, in the process gaining a sense of independence and confidence.

The Unique Challenges of Problem-Solving for Children with DMDD

Children with DMDD often experience emotions with an intensity that can feel allconsuming. This emotional dysregulation and impulsivity can make it challenging for them to engage in reflective, thoughtful problem-solving. Instead, they often react quickly and emotionally, which leads to them making to poor decisions. Witnessing these patterns can be disheartening for parents—their children may struggle to cope with even minor obstacles.

Liam's story illustrates how this difficulty might manifest in everyday life. When faced with a challenging math problem at school, Liam would throw his pencil and refuse to continue, saying he couldn't do it. His frustration quickly turned into anger—he often ripped up his paper and would grab anything he could to throw at the teacher or another student. Not surprisingly, this resulted in frequent trips to the principal's office. His teachers and parents found that Liam was capable of solving math problems when he was calmer, but that when he was faced with a challenge, his immediate emotional reaction created a mental block. When this occurred, his frustration and helplessness triggered a response that escalated into disruptive behavior.

For children like Liam, learning to break down problems into manageable steps can help reduce the anxiety they feel when faced with challenges. Because the sense of being overwhelmed is common in children with DMDD, the first step in teaching them how to problem-solve is to help them identify the problem they're attempting to solve.

Step 1: Identify the Problem

This is a crucial initial step, because children with DMDD often react emotionally to situations without fully understanding what's triggering their distress. A well-defined problem allows children to focus their attention on how best to begin finding a solution.

Parents play a crucial role in guiding their children through the process of articulation. This involves asking questions to help the child break down what's happening and why it feels overwhelming. For example, if a child is upset about a situation at school, a parent might say, "It seems like you're feeling frustrated about what happened today. Can you tell me what you feel made you so upset?" If the child says "I don't know," a parent can turn it into a problem-solving task by asking "When did you get upset?" or offering the following statement: "Sometimes we don't know what upsets us, but maybe we can figure it out."

These types of questions encourage the child to reflect on the specific issue rather than react to the situation's overall emotional weight. It also models the importance of identifying the root cause of a problem before jumping to solutions.

For parents like Raj and Priya, witnessing their child's progress in problem-solving can bring a sense of relief and hope. When Anika came home angry after having been excluded from a group activity at school, Raj and Priya used the strategy of articulation to guide her through the situation. Instead of focusing on her anger, they gently encouraged her to explain what had happened step by step. As Anika described the situation, they could help her see that her peers' actions were hurtful, and they could also guide her to explore why her peers had excluded her and how she could handle similar situations in the future. This approach helped Anika clarify her problem and calmed her by giving structure to an otherwise overwhelming emotional experience.

Step 2: Brainstorm Solutions

Once the problem has been identified, the next step is generating potential solutions. Children with DMDD may struggle with flexibility in their thinking and may often feel like there's only one correct answer to a problem. Encouraging them to think creatively and develop multiple possible solutions fosters flexibility, and it also reduces the pressure they may feel to get things "right" the first time. Parents can model this process by suggesting various solutions, from practical to creative. For instance, if a child is upset because they don't want to do their homework, the parent could ask, "What are some different things we could do to help make homework time easier for you?" In Liam's case, when her son was unable to provide an answer, Sarah offered several possibilities. She asked him, "Would you like to do your problems one at a time with a small break in between, or would you like to complete them all at once and get them done faster?" She would also ask if he wanted to sit as his desk to do his homework or at the kitchen table. One question she found very helpful was, "Would you like me to help you work through the problem, or should I check your answer after you're done?"

While children may initially have difficulty considering various options to manage a problem, by gaining experience with brainstorming, they have an opportunity to learn that there's often more than one way to solve a problem. This helps reduce anxiety and encourages experimentation with different approaches.

When Maya struggled to get ready for school on time, David and Elena helped her devise different strategies to address the problem. Together, they considered several options: Maya could pack her backpack the night before, set her clothes out, or even create a morning checklist to help her stay on track. Maya found that setting out her clothes before bedtime worked best for her, and overall, the process of brainstorming solutions helped her feel more in control of her mornings. Particularly for children with DMDD, this sense of control and empowerment is a key benefit of learning problem-solving skills.

Step 3: Weigh the Pros and Cons

After generating a list of potential solutions, it's essential to teach children to evaluate the pros and cons of each option. This kind of critical thinking helps children anticipate the outcomes of their decisions and make more thoughtful choices. It also reduces the likelihood of making impulsive decisions that are often driven by immediate emotions rather than long-term consequences.

Parents can guide this process by assisting their children to think through the benefits and drawbacks of each solution. For example, when Anika was deciding whether to confront her peers about being excluded, her parents helped her weigh the potential outcomes, asking, "If you talk to them about how you felt, what would you like to say to them?" After helping Anika with what to say, they could then consider how her friends might respond and how she might handle their different responses. Raj and Priya could also ask Anika how she thought she would feel if she *didn't* say anything. These kinds of questions help create a problem-solving mindset and teach children to think critically and to understand that every decision has consequences. It provides them with the tools to pause and reflect before acting, which is especially important for children with DMDD since they often act impulsively when they feel emotional.

Step 4: Implement the Decision

Once a decision is made, the next step is helping children implement their chosen solution. This step involves planning, follow-through, and monitoring the effectiveness of the decision. For children with DMDD, it's essential to encourage them to persist as they might be tempted to give up if the solution doesn't work immediately or perfectly.

Liam's parents worked with him to implement a strategy for handling his frustration with math. After brainstorming different approaches, Liam decided to take a short break whenever he started feeling frustrated and then return to the problem after calming down. His parents supported him by reminding him about his plan and encouraging him to keep trying even when the first solution didn't work perfectly.

Step 5: Monitor and Reflect on the Outcome

After implementing a decision, parents and children need to reflect on the outcome. Did the solution work as intended? What went well and what could be improved next time? This step is crucial for nurturing resilience and teaching children that problem-solving is not always linear. For children with DMDD, this is particularly valuable because it shifts their mindset from seeing a decision as "right" or "wrong" to viewing it as a learning experience.

Parents can facilitate this reflection by asking open-ended questions and encouraging their child to evaluate the outcome without judgment. For instance, after Liam tried his new strategy for managing frustration during math, his parents could ask, "How did it feel to take a break when you started getting frustrated? Did it help you concentrate better when you returned to the problem?" Questions like this guide children in analyzing what worked and why while also reinforcing that it's okay to tweak their approach if things don't go perfectly.

Maya's parents followed up after she decided to set out her clothes the night before. They noticed that while this strategy helped her mornings run more smoothly, there were still days when she rushed out the door without breakfast. Together, they reflected on this issue and decided to adjust their plan by setting the breakfast table the night before, further reducing their morning stress. This reflective process helped Maya see that adjustments are part of problemsolving, not failures.

> My daughter was frequently late to her elementary school despite waking up an hour and a half before school started. Micromanaging her gave her extreme anxiety. We needed to find a way to help her be more productive while allowing her to control her routine. Finding misplaced shoes, deciding what outfit to wear, setting out her toothbrush and toothpaste, and setting her backpack by the front door the night before helped create a smoother routine. She arrived at school on time immediately, feeling much more in control and in a better mood.

The key is to view reflection as a significant way to promote a growth mindset. Rather than focusing on what went wrong, the conversation should highlight what can be learned from the experience and how it can inform future problem-solving. This helps children perceive setbacks as opportunities for growth, a perception that's integral for building resilience in anyone but especially in children prone to frustration and emotional outbursts. Problem-solving and decision-making skills are essential components of a resilient mindset.

Step 6: Reinforce Independence and Confidence

As children with DMDD develop problem-solving and decision-making skills, parents must gradually help them become more independent by encouraging their children to think about ways of solving problems on their own. That allows children to become more autonomous as they become more adept at handling challenges. This process can be incredibly empowering for children with DMDD, who often feel a lack of control over their environment due to their emotional dysregulation.

Maya, for instance, thrived once her parents began giving her more responsibility in her morning routine. By allowing her to implement her own solutions, Maya improved her organizational skills and developed greater confidence in her ability to manage her day. Her parents continued to offer support, but they made sure that Maya understood that ownership of the routine belonged to her.

This shift can be difficult for parents, especially when their child has struggled with impulsivity or poor decision-making in the past. However, allowing children to experience both the successes and the occasional missteps of their decisions is a key part of their growth. While parents can remain available as guides and support systems, they should resist the urge to intervene too quickly. Children learn best by doing! Their confidence will grow as they successfully navigate problems on their own.

Practical Exercises for Problem-Solving and Decision-Making

To help parents apply these concepts in daily life, this section offers a series of practical exercises that can reinforce problem-solving and decision-making skills in children with DMDD. These exercises are designed to be simple, engaging, and adaptable to different situations. They can be practiced in structured settings like family meetings or during informal moments throughout the day. But a caveat: problem-solving strategies will *not* be effective if parents attempt to implement them when a child is having an emotional meltdown. The incident can be discussed once the child is calm.

Exercise 1: The Decision-Making Jar

This exercise helps children understand that there are often multiple solutions to any problem. Parents can create a decision-making jar filled with slips of paper, each containing a different scenario that the child might encounter:
- "You're upset because you can't find your favorite toy."
- "Your friend doesn't want to play the game you want to play."
- "You spilled juice on the table."

During family time, the child picks a scenario from the jar and the family discusses the problem together. Each person suggests at least one solution and then everyone weighs the pros and cons of each solution. This exercise encourages flexible thinking and lets children see that problems can be approached differently.

To take this a step further, parents can encourage the child to choose one of the proposed solutions and role-play how they would implement it. This helps the child visualize their steps and consider how the solution might play out in real life.

Exercise 2: The Problem-Solving Chart

A problem-solving chart can be a visual tool for children who need help staying organized during decision-making. Parents and children can create the chart together, listing each step of the problem-solving process along the way. The chart might include the following sections:

1. Identify the problem: What is the challenge I'm facing?
2. Brainstorm solutions: What are some different ways I could solve it?
3. Weigh the pros and cons: What might happen if I chose each option?
4. Make a decision: Which option do I think is best?
5. Reflect on the outcome: Did it work? What could I do differently next time?

The chart can be displayed in a common area, such as the kitchen or family room, and children can refer to it whenever they encounter a problem. Parents of younger children might walk them through each step, while older children can use the chart more independently.

This tool provides a structure for decision-making and gives children a sense of accomplishment as they work through each step. Over time, they can internalize and use this process without the chart, building their autonomy and confidence.

Exercise 3: The "What If?" Game

The "What if?" game encourages children to think creatively about potential solutions and consequences. Parents can present a hypothetical scenario and ask their child, "What if we tried this?" The child then explores the potential outcomes of each suggestion. For example:

Scenario: "You lost your homework assignment."

- What if you ask the teacher for a new copy?
- What if you tell your teacher you forgot it?
- What if you make up your assignment tomorrow?

The goal is not to find the answers immediately but to help the child practice thinking through different possibilities and their outcomes. Parents can gently guide the conversation by asking questions that prompt deeper reflection, such as, "What do you think your teacher might say if you told them you forgot your homework?"

This game is effective for children who struggle with impulsivity, as it encourages them to pause and think before acting.

Exercise 4: The Emotion Thermometer

The Emotion Thermometer exercise helps children with DMDD learn to recognize and regulate their emotions before they become overwhelming. Parents can create a visual "thermometer" with different levels of intensity, from calm to highly upset, and label each level with emotions like "calm," "frustrated," "angry," and "explosive."

When the child starts to feel upset, parents can encourage them to identify where they are on the thermometer and talk about what emotions they're experiencing. For example, the child might say, "I feel like I'm frustrated right now." Parents can then help the child think of strategies to bring their emotions back down to a calmer level, such as deep breathing, taking a break, or talking about their feelings.

This exercise helps children become more aware of their emotional states and equips them with tools they need to manage their emotions before they escalate. Over time, children may be able to use the thermometer independently, empowering them to regulate their feelings and develop emotional resilience.

Common Obstacles to Problem-Solving and Decision-Making

While teaching problem-solving and decision-making is essential, it's important to recognize that children with DMDD may face unique obstacles that make these processes more challenging. In this section, we'll explore some of the most common roadblocks and provide strategies for overcoming them.

Obstacle 1: Emotional Overload

One of the most significant obstacles for children with DMDD is the intensity of their emotions. When a child is in the middle of an emotional outburst, thinking clearly or considering different options can be nearly impossible—their brain is flooded with emotions, rendering rational problem-solving extremely difficult.

To address this obstacle, parents should focus on emotional regulation before problemsolving. Techniques such as deep breathing, taking a break, or engaging in a calming activity can help the child regain control of their emotions. Only after the child has calmed down should they be encouraged to revisit the problem and consider solutions.

Liam's parents found that allowing him to take short calm-down breaks ahead of attempting his homework significantly improved his ability to concentrate and solve problems. Giving him time to cool off removed the emotional roadblock and made room for clearer thinking. His parents also made sure that Liam had a snack before starting his homework to prevent him from getting hangry—then he could better tackle his assignments.

Obstacle 2: Perfectionism

As noted in Chap. 8, some children (especially those with high anxiety) may struggle with perfectionism, which can hinder their ability to make decisions. They may fear making choices, leading to indecision, or they may avoid the problem altogether.

Parents can help by reassuring their children that often there's no perfect solution to a problem. That makes it okay to make mistakes. Encouraging a growth mindset—where mistakes are seen as learning opportunities—can alleviate the pressure of perfectionism. For instance, parents might say, "It's okay if the solution doesn't work. We can always try something different next time."

This kind of reassurance helps children feel more comfortable experimenting with different approaches and making decisions without fear of failure.

Obstacle 3: Impulsivity

Impulsivity is a common issue for children with DMDD—it makes it difficult for them to pause and think through their decisions. Instead of carefully considering their options, they might react quickly, driven by their emotions or immediate desires. This frequently leads to poor decision-making as the child prioritizes short-term relief over long-term consequences.

To help children manage their impulsivity, parents can introduce a "pause and think" strategy. This involves teaching children to recognize when they're about to make an impulsive decision and gives them tools to pause before acting. One simple technique is "decision child," where the child must wait for a moment before deciding. This slight pause allows them to regain control over their emotions and think through their choices.

Maya's parents had success with this strategy when Maya struggled with impulsivity during playdates. If her friend wanted to play a game she didn't like, she would often react by storming off or demanding they play her way. Her parents taught her to count to five before responding—that helped her take a breath, think about the situation, and react more calmly. Though she sometimes still struggled, pausing before responding began to make a noticeable difference in her interactions with friends.

Obstacle 4: Lack of Confidence

Some children with DMDD may lack confidence in their ability to make good decisions. Because they've experienced frequent emotional outbursts or made impulsive choices that led to adverse outcomes, they might begin to doubt their ability to solve problems independently. This can lead to indecision or relying on others to make decisions for them.

Parents can help by providing opportunities for their children to practice decision-making in low-stakes situations. For example, letting their child choose what to wear from two possible selections, what snack to have, or which game to play bolsters their sense of control and reinforces their ability to make decisions. Positive reinforcement is critical here: when the child makes a decision, even a small one, parents should praise their effort and celebrate the outcome regardless of whether it was the perfect choice. (Obviously, parents should not offer a choice that they would find difficult to accept.)

Liam's lack of confidence in his math skills contributed to his outbursts when he tried to do his homework. His parents started to give him choices about how he approached his homework—for example, whether to tackle the most challenging problems first or leave them for last. This practice slowly built his confidence by allowing him to make these decisions and supporting him regardless of the outcome. Liam began to trust his problem-solving abilities, reducing his frustration and increasing his willingness to tackle complex tasks.

Building Resilience Through Problem-Solving

The ability to solve problems and make sound decisions is closely linked to resilience. Children who can confidently navigate challenges and setbacks are better equipped to handle the emotional ups and downs that come with DMDD. While teaching these skills may take time and patience, the long-term benefits are invaluable.

As children learn to solve problems, they also learn to trust themselves. They begin to understand that even when things don't go as planned, they have the power to adjust, try again, and eventually succeed. This sense of agency is essential for children with DMDD, who often feel overwhelmed by their emotions and circumstances. By giving them the tools to tackle problems independently, parents empower their children to take control of their lives and develop a resilient mindset.

Anika struggled with managing her emotions, especially when it involved making decisions. Simple choices like what to wear or eat often led to long tantrums. Her parents initially took a very hands-on approach, frequently stepping in to make decisions for her to avoid the emotional fallout. However, this approach only reinforced Anika's sense of helplessness and dependency.

After learning about the importance of fostering decision-making and problem-solving skills in children with DMDD, Raj and Priya decided to change their approach. They started small, offering Anika two choices for breakfast instead of deciding for her. At first, this led to frustration on Anika's part—she found it challenging to choose and often demanded a third option. However, with consistent encouragement, Anika slowly began to engage in decision making.

To further support Anika's development, her parents introduced a problem-solving chart to help her manage more complex decisions. When she had difficulty deciding how to handle a situation with a friend who didn't want to play the same game, Raj and Priya sat down with her and used the chart to work through the problem. They helped her identify the problem (her friend wanted to play a different game), brainstorm solutions (she could suggest taking turns, playing the other game first, or choosing a new game together), and weigh the pros and cons of each option. Using this structured support, the next time this incident occurred, Anika suggested taking turns, and her friend agreed.

This process not only helped Anika cope with the immediate challenge but also gave her a framework for how to make future decisions. She became more confident in her ability to solve problems and her emotional outbursts began to decrease in frequency and intensity. Raj and Priya were amazed at the transformation in their daughter! They felt empowered as parents— they knew they were helping Anika build essential life skills.

Real-Life Applications for Parents

Parents can focus on consistent practice, patience, and support to help their children integrate problem-solving and decision-making skills into their daily lives. The following strategies can be adapted to various situations and age groups:

Encouraging Decision-Making in Everyday Situations

Parents can look for opportunities in everyday life where children can make decisions. Depending on age and maturity, these can range from small, routine choices to more involved ones. For instance, parents can allow children to choose between two snacks, decide which route to take during a walk, or select a family movie for the evening. As a child becomes more comfortable with making decisions, parents can gradually increase the complexity of the choices. They might invite their child to help plan a family meal, pick out their clothing for the day, or even decide how to spend their weekend free time.

> We were planning a family vacation, and our son suggested Legoland in Florida. He learned about the theme park from watching YouTube videos by a family who documented their vacation there. We decided Legoland was a good destination and added a few extra days to visit Disney World. Our son loved Legoland, but Disney was too big and stimulating for him, which made the trip extremely difficult. Later, we realized he knew exactly what to expect in Legoland, right down to the hotel room and rides from watching the videos. We didn't think to have our son research Disney, which, if we had, the trip may have gone more smoothly, despite it being massive, because he would have had a better idea of what to expect.

Normalizing Mistakes to Alleviate Anxiety

Children with DMDD experience intense emotions that can make everyday tasks (including making decisions) feel overwhelming. As noted earlier, one of the common challenges they face is a fear of failure, which can paralyze them when it comes to making choices. This fear stems from anxiety about making potential mistakes, which can lead to being indecisive or avoiding tasks altogether. It's crucial for parents to help their child understand that mistakes are a natural and valuable part of the learning process. By normalizing the idea that not every decision will result in a perfect outcome, parents can reduce the pressure children feel when faced with choices.

If a decision doesn't go as planned, parents can use that as an opportunity to nurture resilience. They can encourage their child to reflect on the experience, focusing on what they can learn rather than dwelling on what went wrong. This can be as simple as asking a child, "What could you try differently next time?" Instead of reinforcing negative self-talk, parents can shift their child's mindset from a fear of failure to one of growth. Over time, children learn that regardless of the outcome, each decision offers valuable insights, and that making mistakes doesn't define their abilities or worth.

Practicing Problem-Solving During Family Discussions

Family meetings and discussions provide excellent opportunities to model and practice problem-solving skills in a real-world context. When a family challenge arises—such as deciding on a vacation destination, managing household chores, or planning a family event—parents should make it a point to include their child in the conversation. They should encourage them to voice their opinions, brainstorm ideas, and suggest solutions even if ultimately the parents make the final decision. Getting children involved teaches them that their input is valued and their thoughts matter, which in fosters a sense of ownership and responsibility within the family unit.

Moreover, by participating in discussions, children learn the importance of teamwork and can observe the process of collaborative decision-making. They observe how problems can be approached from multiple angles, how to weigh pros and cons, and how compromises can be made for the greater good of the family. This practice not only helps build their confidence but also strengthens their problem-solving abilities, preparing them for more complex decisions in the future. Additionally, it reinforces the notion that challenges can be handled together, promoting a sense of unity and cooperation within the family.

Using Visual Aids and Tools

Visual aids such as problem-solving charts and decision trees can be highly beneficial for children who struggle with abstract thinking or require more structure to process decisions effectively. These tools provide a concrete, organized framework that guides the child through each step of the decision-making process, breaking the overall scenario down into manageable parts. By having a clear visual reference, children can more easily see the connections between their choices, the potential outcomes, and the steps they need to take. Seeing this larger picture helps reduce feelings of being overwhelmed.

For example, Liam often felt anxious when he was making decisions because he tended to overthink possible outcomes. Therefore, when Liam was faced with deciding how to spend his weekend, his parents introduced him to a decision tree. The first branch asked, "Do you want to stay at home or go out?" From there, each option led to further branches, such as "What will you do at home?" or "Where would you like to go?" This visual representation allowed Liam to see his options clearly and weigh them without becoming bogged down in abstract thoughts or anxiety about making the wrong choice.

Using these visual tools not only helps children like Liam feel more in control, it also teaches them how to approach decisions systematically. Over time, they may begin to internalize these steps, becoming more confident in their ability to think through challenges independently. This method transforms decision-making into a structured and less daunting task, empowering children to engage thoughtfully with their choices.

> On the first day of equestrian therapy, my son was in an awful mood even though he had been looking forward to spending time with the horses. The instructor noticed my son's irritability, which was obvious from the moment we arrived. When the instructor had my son place his hands on the horse for a few minutes, my dysregulated son started to relax and appeared to be calm. From there, he spent 30 minutes learning how to brush and feed the horse, and his entire demeanor had been transformed, from grumpy to joyful during that lesson. He was noticeably a different child from when he arrived.

Praising Effort Over Outcomes

When a child makes a decision, parents must praise their effort and thought process even if the result wasn't what they had hoped for or expected. For example, if a child decides to attempt a new way of organizing their toys but it doesn't work, a parent can say, "I'm proud of you! You tried something new and thought about where to put your toys. Let's think about what we could do differently next time." This approach encourages a growth mindset and reinforces the idea that problem-solving is a process, not a one-time event.

The Long-Term Benefits of Teaching Problem-Solving and Decision-Making

As children with DMDD learn to solve problems and make decisions, they not only gain immediate practical skills, they also lay the foundation for a lifelong benefit: the ability to navigate challenges with greater emotional resilience and thoughtfulness is a skill that will serve them well throughout their entire lives. As they grow into adolescence and adulthood, these skills can help them become more successful in facing complex situations, ranging from finding their way through academic pressures and social dynamics to dealing with workplace challenges and personal relationships.

One of the most significant long-term benefits of applying effective problem-solving techniques is improved emotional regulation. By learning how to approach problems systematically, children with DMDD are better equipped to manage intense emotions. This reduces the frequency of their emotional outbursts. Better emotional regulation allows them to build stronger, more stable relationships with peers, family members, and future colleagues. Additionally, as they become more confident in their decision-making, they're more likely to take on new opportunities and confront challenges head-on rather than avoid difficult situations out of fear or frustration.

Parents who invest time and effort in helping their children develop these skills are providing them with a toolkit for independence. These children become adults who are increasingly self-sufficient and proactive in handling stress and managing their own lives. The shift from feeling reactive to feeling in control can greatly enhance their quality of life, fostering success in both personal and professional arenas.

Final Words

Teaching problem-solving and decision-making skills to children with DMDD is both a challenge and an opportunity that requires patience, consistency, and empathy. The structured approach we've outlined—identifying problems, brainstorming solutions, weighing pros and cons, and reflecting on outcomes—not only provides a clear framework for moving forward, it also empowers children to engage in self-regulation and cognitive flexibility. These skills are essential for any child, but particularly for children with DMDD, who may struggle with emotional outbursts and frustration. By breaking down complex tasks into manageable steps, parents and caregivers can create an environment where children feel safe to express themselves and work through their difficulties.

The lives of Maya, Liam, and Anika demonstrate how—with consistent guidance— children can gain better control over their emotions and make decisions that reflect thoughtfulness rather than impulsivity. Each child's unique progress highlights the transformative potential of nurturing problem-solving skills in everyday situations. Whether it's deciding how to handle a conflict with peers or determining the best approach to a school project, these skills provide a foundation for greater independence.

As children develop these abilities, they also cultivate their self-confidence because they know that they possess the tools they need to approach problems with a calm, confident, and measured mindset. This empowerment can lead to improved relationships, better academic performance, and improved overall emotional well-being. Investing in these skills is a lifelong gift!

Chapter 10
Disciplining in Ways that Promote Self-Discipline and Self-Worth

Nathan's Story

Nathan Taylor's story begins in the United Kingdom—he displayed signs of discomfort and distress when he was just a few weeks old. His parents noticed that he was hypersensitive to touch, engaged in dangerous play without noticing injuries, and was often confused when he hurt others. By the time Nathan was three, his destructive behaviors had escalated, leading to his expulsion from nursery school due to violent and uncontrollable outbursts. His parents struggled to understand their son's behavior. His father Stuart shared, "Nathan was exhibiting frequent rages and destruction at home that were often triggered by seemingly minor frustrations."

At four years old, Nathan's pediatrician diagnosed him with autism spectrum disorder (ASD). Unfortunately, his parents noticed that traditional autism strategies only seemed to exacerbate his distress. Desperate for help, they sought a diagnosis of ADHD. Still, the medication trials—including methylphenidate and guanfacine—only worsened his rages. "We reached a crisis point," said Stuart. "Nathan was experiencing multiple daily rages, leaving my wife and me exhausted and feeling hopeless."

Nathan's parents eventually found a highly recommended pediatric psychiatrist who diagnosed Nathan with ADHD and ASD and also introduced his parents to the concept of DMDD, a relatively new diagnosis in the United Kingdom. This psychiatrist warned them of the severe nature of Nathan's psychiatric problems and encouraged them to fight for his care. They did. But despite their efforts (which included trying various ADHD medications and antipsychotics), nothing seemed to help.

The turning point came when Stuart discovered an online lecture by Dr. Larry Fisher, who described DMDD in a way that perfectly matched Nathan's behaviors. Then the Taylors learned about the Matthews Protocol. Despite skepticism from others, Nathan's parents decided to pursue this treatment privately, as it was not available through the National Health Service. "The protocol brought profound changes for Nathan," said Stuart. "His rages—which were daily occurrences—became rare and less intense. His overall distress reduced significantly, allowing him to engage more in dialogue and respond to calming strategies." The strategies that had failed to help before had finally worked.

While the protocol required them to pay for the medications privately, Nathan's parents strongly believed that the transformation in their son's behavior was worth the cost. For the first time, they felt they had found a truly effective treatment that worked, giving them hope for a more stable and peaceful future for their son. Having achieved stability for the first time, Nathan became more receptive to being taught by his parents in ways that provided him with discipline and promoted his self-worth instead of punitive methods that had failed in the past and had worked *against* his self-esteem. Now that he was stable and less reactive, therapy could finally help Nathan.

The topic of discipline generates significant debate among parents, teachers, and childcare specialists, especially when managing children with mental health challenges such as DMDD. In our workshops and clinical practice, one of the most frequently asked questions revolves around how to discipline children effectively. Every parent seems to have encountered conflicting advice, whether from books, mental health professionals, or their own upbringing. The challenge is even greater for parents raising children with DMDD, who often experience intense irritability, frequent mood swings, and difficulty with regulating their emotions. All of those behaviors complicate the process of implementing traditional discipline strategies.

> The first time my son raged, he was nine years old. We had just switched his stimulant for ADHD to a different brand because he maxed out on the dose. He was 65 pounds, yet his strength was fierce during the rages. His eyes widened, and his face looked different. He was screaming, throwing large objects at my husband and me, flipping the furniture, and taking the mattress off his bed. He was spitting in my husband's face, biting my arm, and hitting us both. It was the first time we ever heard him growl like an animal. It was a frightening experience that lasted for two hours. When he finally calmed down, he didn't remember any of it. Although we had been dealing with chronic irritability and frequent meltdowns, we had never experienced the intensity and duration of a rage. From that night on, our lives had changed, and our son's rages would become frequent. He was quickly pulled off the stimulant as we learned that stimulants magnify underlying mood disorders. After a misdiagnosis of pediatric-onset bipolar, our son was eventually diagnosed with DMDD.

The extreme emotional fluctuations that children with DMDD experience significantly influence their mindsets about discipline—such emotional highs and lows can make it incredibly difficult for them to connect their behavior with the consequences that follow. For example, when a child with DMDD has an explosive outburst due to frustration, they may be so overwhelmed by their emotional response that they cannot recognize or appreciate the causeand-effect relationship between their actions and any disciplinary consequences they receive. Essentially, the intensity of the child's emotions in that moment often clouds their ability to process the situation rationally, making it more difficult for them to link their behavior to what happens afterward.

This disconnection is rooted in the neurological and emotional dysregulation common in children with DMDD. During heightened emotional states, their brains are flooded with stress hormones, limiting their capacity for logical thinking and problem-solving. As a result, when parents or caregivers attempt to discipline them, children with DMDD may not appreciate the connection between their behavior and the discipline being applied, such as losing a privilege or receiving a timeout. Instead, they may view the consequence as unfair or unrelated, further fueling their emotional dysregulation. This makes traditional disciplinary strategies—which rely on a clear understanding of cause and effect—particularly challenging for these children.

When a child with DMDD is in a heightened emotional state, that doesn't just affect their body and mind, it also creates challenges for their parents, who are trying to help their child navigate their intense feelings. But when their child is upset, their body goes into overdrive, making it extremely difficult for them to calm down or reason. It's not that the child doesn't want to behave or listen—the problem is that their brain and body are overwhelmed by emotions and the chemical rush that takes over everything.

One of the key players in this reaction is the vagus nerve. The vagus nerve is a crucial part of the parasympathetic nervous system, extending from the brain to the heart, lungs, and digestive tract. It helps regulate involuntary functions like heart rate and digestion, and it calms the body after stress; essentially, the vagus nerve plays a key role in emotional and physical responses. For a child with DMDD, it struggles to operate efficiently, and as a result, a child may stay in a heightened state for much longer, making it seem like they're overreacting or being defiant when in reality they're stuck in an emotional "high gear." This can be highly frustrating for parents, who may feel like nothing they do is helping their child regain control.

When emotions run high, the body releases chemicals like adrenaline and cortisol. These chemicals make the child's heart race, their muscles tense, and their mind hyper alert. While the child is in this state, trying to reason with them or asking them to calm down can feel impossible. For parents, this often feels like a losing battle—they may try to impose discipline, but the child is too emotionally charged to respond in a way that seems reasonable. This can lead to cycles of frustration where both the parent and the child feel stuck, unable to break free from the swirl of intense emotions.

As these emotional episodes continue, the child's ability to develop self-discipline can be affected, because when a child is constantly in a heightened state, learning how to manage their emotions becomes harder. Self-discipline relies on the ability to pause, reflect, and make choices, but for a child with DMDD, this process is interrupted by the flood of stress hormones that make it difficult to slow down and think clearly. Instead, their brain is often more focused on surviving the emotional storm than learning from it.

This can be heartbreaking for parents. They want to teach their child how to control their emotions, but it feels as if the child can't get there no matter what they try. Over time, the parent and child may feel exhausted by these repeated emotional battles, which can significantly strain the relationship. Parents might feel unsure about how to discipline their child in a way that helps rather than makes things worse, while children may feel discouraged because they can't gain control of their feelings.

Fortunately, understanding what's happening inside the child's body can help. Knowing that the child isn't intentionally being difficult but is physically and emotionally overwhelmed can shift how parents approach discipline. Instead of focusing on punishment, the goal becomes helping the child learn to calm down and manage their emotions—only then can discipline be effective. Techniques like moving to a quiet, safe space to cool down, engaging in deep breathing, or practicing mindfulness can support the vagus nerve and help the child escape their heightened state. Over time, with the proper support and often medication, children with DMDD can start to develop self-discipline, but reaching that goal requires patience, understanding, and using strategies that focus on calming the body and mind first. Although this journey can be challenging for both parents and children, with time, understanding, and the right approach, it *is* possible to help children with DMDD develop healthier emotional regulation and better self-discipline.

Again, though, it's critical for parents to understand what's happening to their child during their outbursts. Experiencing such emotional extremes often leads to a feeling of helplessness or victimization for anyone, and when a child is unable to regulate their emotions, they may perceive discipline not as a natural consequence of their behavior but as an unpredictable or even punitive response from their caregiver. This perception can erode the child's trust in the disciplinary process, making them more likely to act out in future situations because they don't see the consequences imposed upon them as being an opportunity for learning and growth. Therefore, parents must adopt a disciplined approach that's more focused on emotional guidance and regulation than just punitive consequences. Doing so helps bridge the gap between behavior and understanding the consequences of that behavior.

Anika's mother once explained her frustration with respect to discipline, saying, "I've tried everything with Anika: timeouts, reasoning, rewards, consequences, even raising my voice when I get frustrated. But nothing seems to stick. I know I'm not supposed to yell, but when I don't, she just ignores me." Her experience echoes the sentiments of many parents—so many feel adrift and unsure of what to do when it comes to disciplining their children.

This chapter focuses on discipline strategies that foster self-discipline and self-worth, crucial components of resilience and emotional regulation for children with DMDD. The goal is to provide guidance that helps children like Anika, Liam, and Maya develop healthier behaviors while maintaining a positive sense of self and nurturing their emotional growth. These strategies aim to create an environment where the child feels supported, understood, and empowered to make better behavioral choices over time.

The Role of Discipline in Building Resilience

When viewed as a teaching process, discipline is essential for helping children develop resilience, which is the ability to manage adversity effectively. The word "discipline" comes from the Latin word "discipline," meaning "instruction" or "training," and is closely related to the word "disciple," which refers to someone who learns from a teacher or guide. In this context, discipline should be seen as an educational tool rather than simply a method of enforcing obedience. Its purpose is not just to stop undesirable behavior but to teach children how to manage their emotions, behaviors, and choices in a more constructive and regulated manner.

Consider Liam, a child who frequently experienced explosive outbursts when he felt frustrated or overwhelmed. Liam's reactions may have seemed disproportionate to the situation at hand, but they reflected his difficulty in processing and regulating his emotions. If Liam's parents had responded to his outbursts with punitive measures like yelling or punishment, that might have escalated his distress and caused him to feel even more out of control. The key to disciplining Liam effectively was not simply to stop the outburst in the moment—instead, his parents needed to provide discipline either afterward or during calmer moments when his brain was able to process words and concepts more clearly. This approach helped him understand and manage the emotions that were driving his behavior.

In Liam's case, discipline was not just about enforcing consequences for bad behavior, it was about teaching him to recognize his emotions and offering him tools to regulate them. When Liam got frustrated, his parents sometimes guided him through calming techniques like deep breathing and sometimes encouraged him to take a break when he started to feel overwhelmed. The goal was for Liam to gradually develop the internal mechanisms that would allow him to manage his own behavior even when his parents or caregivers weren't immediately there to guide him.

Shifting the Focus: From Punishment to Emotional Growth

For parents of children with DMDD, the biggest challenge often lies in shifting the focus from traditional punitive discipline to strategies that promote emotional intelligence and resilience. To discipline effectively in a way that fosters long-term resilience, parents must approach discipline with empathy, consistency, and clear communication. For example, instead of reacting to Liam's outbursts with frustration, his parents acknowledged his emotions by saying, "I see you're really upset right now. Let's take a moment to calm down, and then we can figure this out together." This response showed empathy for his emotional state while also setting a boundary that he needed to calm down before they could continue the conversation.

Consistency is another critical component of building resilience through discipline because children with DMDD need predictable responses to their behavior. To once again use Liam as an example, if he knew that his parents would respond calmly and consistently each time he had an outburst, that surety created a sense of security for him. He learned that his emotional outbursts would not be met with unpredictability or anger but with support and guidance, an expectation that helped him feel safer in working through his emotions.

Developing Emotional Intelligence and Problem-Solving Skills

One of the primary goals of discipline should be to help children develop emotional intelligence. That includes the ability to recognize, understand, and manage their emotions as well as to recognize and respond to the emotions of others. For children with DMDD, emotional intelligence is particularly important because it allows them to navigate their intense emotional experiences more effectively.

Michael and Sarah were able to encourage Liam to develop his emotional intelligence by helping him identify and label his emotions—whenever Liam began to feel frustrated, they would say something like, "It looks like you're feeling frustrated because this task is hard. Let's figure out how we can make it easier." Such responses not only validated his feelings but also taught him to recognize frustration as a specific emotion that he could address. Over time, Liam began to recognize his own emotional triggers and apply the strategies he had learned to manage them.

Similarly, problem-solving skills are another key component of resilience. As discussed in Chap. 9, when children with DMDD encounter challenges—whether it's a difficult task at school or a disagreement with a friend—they need tools to work through the situation in a constructive way. In Liam's case, rather than stepping in to solve the problem for him, his parents guided him through the process of identifying the problem, brainstorming potential solutions, and deciding on the best course of action. This step-by-step approach taught Liam that while he might not be able to control every situation, he could learn to control how he could respond to it.

Building a Resilient Mindset

A resilient mindset is characterized by flexibility, problem-solving abilities, the ability to function well in the face of adversity, and the capacity to manage setbacks. For children with DMDD, developing this mindset is essential because it helps them cope with the emotional and behavioral challenges they face daily. Parents, for their part, can help their children build a resilient mindset that will serve them well throughout their lives by focusing on teaching rather than punishing. With that kind of guidance, children will begin to understand that setbacks and frustrations are a natural part of life—they do not have to define anyone. Children can learn that they have the ability to regulate their emotions, solve problems, and move forward in a positive direction.

In the long term, taking this kind of approach to discipline not only supports children with DMDD in the moment, but it also lays the foundation for healthy interpersonal relationships and success in various aspects of life, including school, friendships, and eventually the workplace. Children who develop resilience through effective discipline are more likely to approach challenges with confidence, perseverance, and a belief in their ability to overcome obstacles.

Discipline as a Foundation for Resilience

When discipline is viewed as an educational process rather than a punishment, it becomes a powerful tool for teaching children how to manage their emotions, behaviors, and choices in a way that promotes long-term well-being. For children with DMDD, the goal of discipline is not simply to stop an undesirable behavior but to guide them toward self-regulation and emotional growth.

By shifting the focus from punitive measures to strategies that build emotional intelligence and problem-solving skills, parents can help their children develop the resilience they need to face life's challenges with confidence and flexibility. This approach encourages children to reflect on their actions, understand the consequences of their choices, and learn from their mistakes in a constructive way. Parents become mentors in helping their children cultivate essential life skills like patience, empathy, and responsibility. Over time, these qualities foster a sense of autonomy and self-efficacy, ensuring that children are not only prepared to thrive in their relationships and personal endeavors but also to navigate the complexities of the adult world with emotional maturity and strength.

Understanding DMDD and the Role of Discipline

Children diagnosed with DMDD frequently exhibit extreme irritability, anger, and temper outbursts. This is not a sign of defiance but rather a reflection of a child's difficulty in regulating their emotions. These children don't simply need stricter rules or more discipline—their emotional regulation systems are wired differently, and traditional disciplinary methods like timeouts or punishments can often exacerbate the problem.

Maya's parents, for instance, shared their struggles in handling her emotional outbursts. "We tried to put her in timeout whenever she had a meltdown, but instead of calming down, she would scream louder and throw things," said Priya. "We were at a loss." This is a common experience for parents of children with DMDD, unfortunately. Punitive approaches often backfire because they don't address the underlying emotional dysregulation and can instead increase the child's frustration, making their behavior worse.

For children like Maya, effective discipline must focus on prevention and understanding the triggers that lead to outbursts. Rather than reacting to her behavior with punishment, her parents needed to learn to identify the situations or emotions that caused her meltdowns. Discipline in the context of DMDD must prioritize teaching coping strategies (i.e., deep breathing or taking a break) and providing consistent and clear boundaries. Parents must also approach discipline as a learning opportunity—they need to validate their child's emotions and discuss solutions together rather than frame disciplining their child as a power struggle.

Positive Reinforcement: Building on Strengths

One of the most effective tools in disciplining children with DMDD is positive reinforcement. This method involves recognizing and rewarding desirable behaviors, helping the child understand what's expected of them, and encouraging them to repeat desirable behaviors. For children who often feel out of control due to their emotional dysregulation, positive reinforcement can provide them with a sense of mastery over their environment. This perception is essential for developing self-discipline.

In Liam's case, by focusing on acknowledging and rewarding positive behaviors rather than punishing negative ones, Michael and Sarah were able to shift the tone of discipline in their home. Instead of being constantly reactive, they became proactive in reinforcing the behaviors they wanted to see more of from Liam. This approach helped Liam feel proud of his accomplishments, which in turn encouraged him to continue developing his emotional regulation skills.

Implementing Positive Reinforcement

A positive feedback system can be customized to a child's specific needs and interests. For example, parents can offer encouraging comments to help their child calm down after feeling upset, complete chores without being reminded, and peacefully resolve conflicts with a sibling. This kind of positive reinforcement must be specific and immediate so that children will more easily understand the connections between their behavior and positive feedback. For instance, if a child takes a deep breath instead of yelling, their parent should immediately acknowledge and praise this effort, saying, "I'm proud of how you took a deep breath instead of yelling." This immediate feedback helps reinforce the behavior and encourages the child to continue using the skill in the future.

It's also important to celebrate small victories. While children with DMDD may not make significant progress overnight, even small steps toward emotional regulation should be recognized and celebrated. Each step forward, no matter how small, is a sign that the child is learning and growing, and celebrating these moments can reinforce their sense of accomplishment and self-worth.

Consistency in Rules and Expectations

Children with DMDD thrive in environments where rules and expectations are clear, consistent, and predictable. Consistency gives them a sense of security and control, and that can reduce anxiety and minimize emotional outbursts. For Anika, inconsistency in routines— especially around bedtime—was a major trigger for meltdowns. Her mother shared that they struggled to enforce a bedtime routine. "One night we let her stay up because she was upset, and then the next night we tried to enforce an early bedtime. That led to a huge tantrum," Priya explained. "It felt like we were constantly walking on eggshells, unsure of what would set her off."

In this case, Anika needed clear and consistent rules about bedtime that were not subject to change based on her emotional state. When parents are consistent with their expectations, children know what to expect and they feel more in control. This is especially important for children with DMDD, who can feel overwhelmed by unpredictable environments. That kind of feeling often leads to increased dysregulation.

Implementing consistency requires establishing routines for key parts of the day, such as mealtimes, bedtimes, and transitions from one activity to another. Sticking to these routines as much as possible helps create an environment in which children feel safe and know what's expected of them. However, it's also important to be firm but flexible when necessary. For example, if a child is having an exceptionally difficult day, their parents might explain why the rule is being adjusted for that moment, but they must also emphasize that this is an exception, *not* a new rule.

For younger children or those who struggle with verbal communication, using visual aids like charts or schedules can help reinforce consistency. A visual schedule allows the child to see what's coming next, reducing anxiety about transitions and helping them prepare for upcoming activities. By clearly outlining daily expectations, visual aids can prevent many misunderstandings and reduce the likelihood of emotional meltdowns.

Six Strategies for Promoting Self-Discipline

Emotional Regulation Before Consequence-Based Discipline

Emotional regulation is the foundation upon which meaningful discipline is built, especially for children with conditions like DMDD. These children experience emotions so intensely that without proper regulation, they struggle to connect their actions to consequences. Therefore, teaching self-soothing strategies—deep breathing, counting to ten, taking a break—is crucial. These techniques provide children with the ability to calm their bodies and minds. Only when the child is more relaxed can they begin to reflect on their actions and understand why certain behaviors are inappropriate. By prioritizing emotional regulation first, parents set the stage for more effective discipline, leading to long-term behavioral improvement.

Priya also found that incorporating soothing music helped calm her daughter, making her more open to a productive discussion about her behavior. After a tantrum, Priya would turn on Anika's favorite calming playlist while assisting her to breathe slowly. Combining familiar music and deep breathing helped Anika regain control over her emotions, making the conversation about her actions more successful and less aggressive. Parents must keep in mind that some children are just not willing or able to have a discussion about their behavior immediately following an outburst—it may take them a while to get there.

> My 14-year-old son refused to get up for school after getting in big trouble the night before. This was rare for him. He was still furious at us and wanted to retaliate over what had transpired by refusing to go to school. If this had been our daughter, who has only ADHD, we could have negotiated in the moment to get her out of bed and to school on time, even with her still angry. But with our son, he needed time to sit in his feelings, accept his consequences, and calm down. Threatening him and pushing him to his breaking point has never been productive, not even to satisfy our desire to get to school on time. Allowing him to sit in his feelings to process them while missing a few classes allowed him to calm down and have a thoughtful and productive conversation with us. Handling a situation at the moment, unless it is a life-or-death situation, with our DMDD son will almost always lead to escalated emotions and volatility. We would have preferred him not to miss any classes that day, but what was more important was that he could process his emotions and calm down in a safe environment. Having this flexibility usually results in better outcomes.

Consistent Routines to Reduce Anxiety

Because children with DMDD often feel overwhelmed by unpredictability, it's crucial for parents to establish structured routines—predictability in daily life provides these children with a sense of security, which in turn reduces anxiety. Consistent routines also minimize the emotional strain of transitioning between activities, something that often triggers emotional outbursts. Parents can help by creating straightforward, easy-to-follow exercises with visual aids like schedules or checklists. When children with DMDD have a greater sense of control over what will come next, their anxiety levels are lower and they're more likely to be in a calmer, more stable emotional state. All of this reduces the likelihood of meltdowns and frustration throughout the day.

Maya's parents introduced transitional reminders like five-minute alerts before any activity change. For instance, when switching from playtime to dinner, they set a timer that gave her a countdown. This method helped Maya anticipate and accept transitions, minimizing the likelihood of emotional flare-ups and helping her adjust more smoothly to changes in her routine. A related technique is to include a choice with the reminders, such as asking the child if they would like the parent to let them know four minutes before the transition or six minutes before the transition.

Response Cost: Empowering Children with DMDD to Maintain Positive Behaviors

Response cost is a behavioral strategy that can be particularly effective in helping children with DMDD learn to manage their emotions and behaviors. This approach involves removing a valued item or privilege in response to negative behavior, allowing children to directly experience the consequences of their actions. Rather than focusing on punishment, response cost encourages children to actively work toward keeping what they have, fostering a sense of responsibility and control over their actions.

For children with DMDD, the concept of losing something they value (extra screen time, a favorite toy, a particular activity) due to inappropriate behavior can be a powerful motivator. It shifts the dynamic from punitive discipline to one where the child is empowered to make choices and see the immediate results of their behavior. When used consistently and fairly, response cost helps children understand the connections between their actions and consequences, reinforcing the importance of self-regulation and emotional control.

All that said, in order for response cost to be effective, parents and caregivers must communicate expectations clearly and ensure that the consequences are proportionate to the behavior. Combining response cost with positive reinforcement for good behavior creates a balanced approach and helps children learn to control their emotions while empowering them to make positive choices.

In Maya's case, she often struggled with emotional outbursts when asked to stop doing something she enjoyed, like playing video games. Her parents decided to implement the response cost method to help her manage these emotions. They tied her favorite activity—playing video games after doing her homework—to her behavior. When Maya became upset and yelled when they asked her to stop playing, her parents calmly reminded her that her outburst would cost her 15 minutes of game time the following day.

At first, this frustrated Maya even more—she thought it was unfair to lose something she valued. But Raj and Priya consistently stuck with their approach, and gradually, Maya began to connect the dots between her behavior and the consequences. She began practicing better control over her reactions to preserve her gaming time. With this consistent application of response cost, Maya's emotional outbursts became less frequent, and she also felt more empowered because she knew that her behavior directly influenced her outcomes. The response cost method helped Maya manage her anger and improved her understanding of responsibility and the rewards of emotional regulation.

Meanwhile, Liam consistently resisted bedtime, turning it into a nightly struggle. He would stall by requesting more stories or extra time with his parents and then often had tantrums when he was told it was time to go to bed. In response, Liam's parents introduced the response cost method, with the clear understanding that negative behavior—such as stalling, whining, or defiance—would result in losing story time. One evening, Liam lost five minutes of his story time after he refused to cooperate. Though initially upset, Liam soon realized that his actions directly impacted whether or not he could enjoy his bedtime stories.

Over time, the consistent use of response cost motivated Liam to follow the routine since he didn't want to lose any of his story time. Gradually, his bedtime resistance decreased and he learned to cooperate more smoothly. Michael and Sarah noticed an improvement in his bedtime routine and his emotional regulation as he began to understand that staying calm and cooperative allowed him to keep his privileges. That realization gave him greater control over his behavior.

Empathy and Emotional Validation

Empathy is the cornerstone of any effective discipline strategy, particularly with emotionally sensitive children. Acknowledging and validating a child's feelings builds trust and helps de-escalate emotionally charged situations. When parents show empathy, children feel understood, and that's particularly important for children with DMDD as they often feel isolated or misunderstood in the midst of their emotional intensity. Of course, validating emotions doesn't mean condoning bad behavior! But it does open the door for a more productive conversation. The child is more likely to engage with a parent who understands their emotional state, making it easier to guide them toward appropriate behaviors.

In addition to displaying empathy, Anika's father also used reflective listening, repeating her emotions to ensure that Anika felt heard. That reduced her resistance and calmed her down more quickly. For example, when Anika became upset about not getting ice cream, Raj said, "I see that you're disappointed because you were excited about it." His acknowledgment made her feel understood, so instead of getting more frustrated, she calmed down. Her father was then able to explain why it wasn't the right time for dessert.

A Problem-Solving Approach

Using a problem-solving approach instead of focusing on punishment allows children to develop critical thinking skills they can use throughout their lives. By guiding children through identifying triggers, emotions, and potential solutions, parents help them gain valuable insights into their behavior. This method fosters autonomy and teaches children to manage their feelings and actions independently. Instead of simply reacting to discipline, children learn to reflect and actively participate in finding more effective ways to handle similar situations in the future. This approach encourages collaboration and strengthens children's sense of agency, making them more invested in improving their behavior.

After discussing her meltdowns, Maya's parents helped her identify coping mechanisms she could use, like finding a quiet space. Their conversations gave her a sense of control over the situation. David and Elena also practiced role-playing scenarios at home to allow her to test her new coping skills in a safe, supportive environment. One of those scenarios was pretending to be in a crowded store where Maya used her noise-canceling headphones. Being able to practice her coping skills in advance made Maya feel more confident when she was faced with similar situations in the real world.

Teaching Coping Skills

Teaching coping skills during calmer moments is essential for long-term emotional regulation, especially for children prone to intense emotional reactions. Well-practiced coping skills like deep breathing, visualization, mindfulness, and grounding techniques offer children tangible tools to calm themselves in the heat of the moment. Parents should practice these skills with their children regularly so that they become second nature in stressful situations. By empowering children with these tools, parents help their children become more independent and reduce the frequency and intensity of their emotional outbursts.

Besides counting to ten, Liam's parents introduced him to progressive muscle relaxation, helping him become more aware of how stress affected his body and how to release it. During particularly stressful moments, they would guide him through tensing and relaxing his muscles, starting from his toes and working up to his head. Over time, this routine helped Liam calm down more quickly when he started feeling overwhelmed. This technique prevented many outbursts from escalating.

Obstacles and Solutions in Discipline

Punitive Discipline

Punitive approaches to discipline—especially when they become a tug-of-war between parent and child—often escalate into power struggles. Children with DMDD are especially prone to feeling as though they're being unfairly punished, and they may become defiant and entrenched when they perceive a lack of empathy. This dynamic turns discipline into a battle for control, making it difficult for either party to find a constructive resolution. The child's resistance can intensify the conflict and create a negative feedback loop that worsens the situation rather than diffusing it.

Fortunately, instead of focusing on punitive measures, parents can adopt a more collaborative and growth-oriented approach to discipline. They can engage their child in a problem-solving dialogue by framing discipline as an opportunity for emotional learning rather than a struggle for authority, for example. This shift in perspective encourages the child to take ownership of their behavior and work with their parent to find solutions, in the process fostering their emotional growth. Such an approach reduces the likelihood of resistance and power struggles and makes discipline a shared effort instead of an adversarial confrontation. The child feels supported rather than attacked, which is crucial for emotional development.

The Dangers of Negative Reinforcement

In sharp contrast to positive reinforcement, negative reinforcement—which is often unintentionally employed by parents or caregivers—can exacerbate the emotional and behavioral challenges faced by children with DMDD. When negative behaviors like tantrums, defiance, and outbursts are met with concessions or conflict avoidance, the child may learn that these behaviors achieve the desired outcome. For example, if a child throws a tantrum to avoid doing a task and the task is removed, the negative behavior is reinforced. This creates a cycle where the child learns to use disruptive behavior to manipulate situations, making it increasingly difficult for caregivers to effectively implement discipline.

Negative reinforcement also undermines the development of emotional regulation because children are unintentionally encouraged to rely on emotional outbursts to get what they want instead of learning healthy coping mechanisms or understanding the consequences of their actions. Over time, this pattern can lead to more frequent and intense emotional reactions, further complicating efforts to manage the child's behavior and increasing stress for both the child and the caregiver.

Parents and caregivers must adopt consistent, positive reinforcement strategies to counteract the dangers of negative reinforcement. By rewarding desirable behaviors like calm responses and problem-solving efforts, children learn that positive actions lead to favorable outcomes. Eventually, this approach helps children develop emotional resilience and better selfregulation, reducing the likelihood of emotional outbursts and reinforcing constructive behaviors. Positive reinforcement also fosters a healthier parent-child relationship as it shifts the focus from punishing bad behavior to encouraging and acknowledging good behavior.

Parent Burnout

Parenting a child with DMDD can be emotionally taxing—parents often wind up feeling frustrated when discipline strategies don't seem to be effective. This frustration can build up over time, resulting in reactive disciplinary practices such as yelling, threatening, or issuing harsh punishments. Although these reactions are understandable, they tend to worsen the situation because they increase the child's emotional dysregulation. A parent's frustration may unfortunately cause them to react in ways that further exacerbate the child's stress levels, leading to a cycle of negative interactions that harm the parent-child relationship.

To break this cycle, parents must prioritize their *own* well-being—they must recognize that their own mental health is key to effectively supporting their children. Parents should practice self-care to maintain their emotional resilience, including joining support groups, seeking professional guidance, and/or incorporating mindfulness practices into daily routines. In addition to these resources, parents should consider working with a therapist for their own needs. A personal therapist can provide parents with invaluable support as they navigate the challenges of raising a child, particularly one with DMDD. Therapists can offer strategies to manage stress, maintain a calm and empathetic approach to discipline, and ensure emotional well-being.

These proactive steps helps parents respond to their children with patience and understanding and equip them to handle difficult situations. In particular, when facing external challenges such as interactions with law enforcement or child protective services, having a therapist can provide crucial advocacy and support. This was the case for one parent we spoke with who had successfully navigated a CPS investigation with the help of their therapist.

By getting professional support and taking care of their own emotional health, parents can reduce reactive discipline, create a more supportive environment for their child's emotional development, and enhance their ability to meet their child's needs and the needs of their entire family.

Slow Is Not Fast Enough

For children with DMDD, positive reinforcement may yield little immediate or noticeable changes in behavior. This can make it difficult for parents to continue being patient and persistent. Progress can be slow, and even when positive behaviors are consistently reinforced, it can seem like the child isn't learning or growing. Such a lack of visible improvement may discourage parents and make it more difficult for them to adhere to positive reinforcement techniques. The core challenge lies in recognizing and reinforcing even the most minor signs of progress, as these incremental improvements are part of the child's long-term emotional and behavioral development.

To overcome this challenge, parents should celebrate small victories along the way. *Every* small step forward should be acknowledged and reinforced! These minor achievements are indicators that the child is indeed learning and progressing. Immediate and specific praise is essential to strengthen the desired behavior and encourage the child to continue working on their emotional regulation and self-discipline. By focusing on gradual improvements and acknowledging progress, parents can foster a positive environment in which the child feels motivated to keep trying even when changing takes time. Consistently reinforcing positive behaviors will eventually lead to more lasting improvements.

> As the father of a child with DMDD, I studied biology in college and have always been very health-conscious myself. I'm aware of the gut-brain connection and how some scientists are now considering the gut to be the second brain in many ways. The types and quantity of bacteria in the gut may affect brain chemistry and make one more susceptible to depression, anxiety and mood issues, which was what my son was experiencing. This was a very real possibility, considering that current research supports that 90% of serotonin is produced in the gut. I found some studies that showed that probiotics and prebiotics can positively influence the "gut-brain axis," a complex communication pathway between the gut microbiome and the central nervous system, potentially improving mood, cognitive function, and mental well-being. Adding probiotics and prebiotics to my son's routine was a small thing I could do to help his gut (and brain) be as healthy as possible. I also noticed early on that when my son ate candy loaded with sugar and synthetic dyes it significantly affected his hyperactivity, irritability, and aggression, and those chemicals seemed to stay in his system for a few days. It caused problems with the school because his teachers would frequently use candy to motivate the students. We limit sugar intake at home to prevent a spike and subsequent sharp drop in blood sugar that would inevitably follow and trigger a meltdown. Providing him a diet in whole foods with a focus on protein and healthy fats helps our son be satiated longer and have less sugar cravings between meals.

Hypersensitivity

Children with DMDD are often hypersensitive to their surroundings, making noisy or crowded environments overwhelming. This sensory overload can trigger emotional meltdowns and further complicate efforts to manage the child's behavior. Chaotic environments or those filled with stimuli can feel threatening or confusing to the child, exacerbating their emotional dysregulation and increasing the likelihood of outbursts. Parents may find it challenging to manage the child's behavior in these settings, as the external environment is directly impacting the child's emotional state and making discipline more challenging to implement.

To mitigate this challenge, whenever possible, parents can modify the environment to reduce sensory overload. Creating a calm, quiet space at home can provide children with a safe retreat when they're feeling overwhelmed. Tools like noise-canceling headphones or sensory-friendly toys and fidgets can help children cope with overstimulating environments. Parents can gradually introduce their child to more challenging settings that exist outside the home while teaching them coping strategies like deep breathing or visual cues to manage their emotional responses. With various tools and strategies at their disposal, parents can possibly help prevent meltdowns and create a more manageable atmosphere for their child and for themselves.

Addressing the Underlying Reasons for Challenging Behavior

As we've already discussed, children with DMDD often exhibit challenging behaviors because of underlying emotional needs or triggers. Therefore, understanding and addressing these needs is critical to reduce the frequency and intensity of a child's outbursts. Maya's parents, for instance, discovered that her tantrums were more likely to occur when she felt overwhelmed in crowded or noisy environments. By identifying this pattern, they were able to proactively address the issue. "We started bringing noise-canceling headphones when we went to busy places, and we noticed a huge decrease in her meltdowns," Priya said. "She still got upset sometimes, but it wasn't as explosive."

By identifying the triggers that lead to disruptive behaviors, parents can take steps to prevent certain situations or help their child manage them more effectively. For children like Maya, this might involve modifying the environment—such as providing a quiet space or reducing sensory stimuli—or teaching the child coping strategies to help them manage their emotions when they start to feel overwhelmed.

Tracking behaviors in a behavior journal can be a helpful tool for identifying patterns and triggers. Parents can note the time of day, environment, and specific circumstances surrounding an outburst to assess if there are recurring themes. Over time, this can help parents better anticipate what might trigger a meltdown and they can then adjust their strategies accordingly.

Empathy: The Key to Effective Discipline

As we highlighted in Chap. 4, empathy is a critical dimension of parenting. It's a cornerstone of effective discipline, especially when working with children who have DMDD. These children often feel misunderstood or overwhelmed by their emotions, and when discipline is applied without empathy, the child can be left feeling isolated and unsupported. For instance, when Liam had a meltdown, his mother initially responded with frustration, saying things like "You're too old to be acting this way!" That only escalated the situation, as Liam felt further misunderstood.

After Sarah learned about the power of empathy when it comes to parenting, she drastically changed her approach—instead of trying to stop Liam's behavior immediately, she began by acknowledging and validating his emotions. Whenever Liam was upset, she would say in a calm voice, "I can see you're feeling upset right now. It's okay to feel that way. Let's figure out how to calm down together."

She also became more attuned to his responses during these moments. If she noticed that talking seemed to escalate Liam's distress, she would pause and offer him what he needed most: quiet and space to self-regulate. This subtle but significant shift in her approach helped Liam feel understood rather than punished and fostered a sense of trust and emotional safety.

As a result of Sarah's new tactics, her dynamic with Liam began to change. What was once a cycle of conflict and resistance became opportunities for connection and collaboration. Sarah showed her son that his feelings were valid by leading with empathy, setting the stage for effective problem-solving and mutual understanding. This marked a turning point in their relationship, highlighting the significant impact of responding with care and compassion. When parents practice empathy in discipline, they create an environment where their children feel safe to express their emotions. This approach helps de-escalate tense situations and teaches the child that their feelings are valid and that there are healthy ways to manage them.

Conclusion: Discipline as a Tool for Growth

Disciplining children with DMDD is a complex task. Still, when approached with empathy, consistency, and a focus on positive feedback, it becomes an opportunity to foster emotional and behavioral growth. By helping children understand the underlying reasons for their behavior, offering clear and consistent expectations, and reinforcing positive actions, parents can help their children develop the self-discipline and self-worth they need to thrive. For children with DMDD in particular, learning how to regulate their emotions and behaviors, increase their resilience, and build a more positive sense of self are invaluable lessons as they learn to navigate their emotional world and grow into healthier, more self-assured individuals.

By implementing the strategies outlined in this chapter, parents can assist their children in developing greater self-discipline and resilience. Although it's true that notable obstacles lie along the way, these challenges can be overcome with thoughtful, supportive approaches that address a child's unique emotional needs. Through these strategies, parents can transform discipline from being a source of frustration to becoming a powerful tool for emotional and behavioral growth. With nurturing guidance and patience, children with DMDD can develop the emotional intelligence and resilience they need to thrive in all areas of life, from school settings to social interactions to their future careers.

Chapter 11
Developing Responsibility, Compassion, and a Social Conscience

Ethan's Story

Ethan Tsu is a seven-year-old boy who exhibited frequent emotional outbursts characterized by intense anger and frustration. These episodes would last up to two hours and occurred two to three times per week. Despite these challenges, Ethan demonstrated normal social and academic functioning when he wasn't experiencing an outburst. He was known for his pleasant demeanor and showed no irritability between episodes.

"We were very concerned about Ethan's emotional outbursts not only at home but also at school," said his father David. Eventually, Ethan received a diagnosis of ADHD; his symptoms of impulsivity, hyperactivity, and difficulty focusing were observed in various settings. Ethan's family initially explored the possibility of a diagnosis of DMDD given the severity of his mood swings, but he didn't meet the full diagnostic criteria for DMDD since his emotional regulation issues were less pervasive and didn't involve ongoing irritability outside of his outbursts.

At first, Ethan was prescribed a stimulant medication to manage his ADHD symptoms. That provided some benefits in reducing his hyperactivity and improving his focus. "Unfortunately, we noticed that the medication had only a limited impact on the frequency and severity of Ethan's emotional outbursts, and we felt frustrated," said his mother Amy.

After trying various treatment approaches, Ethan's care team implemented the Matthews Protocol along with a structured behavioral intervention designed to help children with emotional regulation issues. Over time, the Matthews Protocol significantly reduced the frequency, duration, and intensity of Ethan's outbursts. His family and teachers noticed that his episodes became shorter, less severe, and occurred much less frequently, improving Ethan's overall quality of life.

The Matthews Protocol proved to be a turning point in Ethan's treatment—it kept his mood stable, and his ADHD remained well-managed with the stimulant medication. His outbursts were successfully controlled, allowing him to thrive socially and academically. As Ethan's explosive incidents decreased, another key factor in his improvement involved engaging in helping others. This allowed his peers to see Ethan in a new light—instead of being disruptive to the class, he was starting to be viewed in a more positive way. At school, he was given the "job" of holding the door for students to come in after recess. Not only did he feel good about this responsibility, but his job addressed another issue, namely that it had often taken Ethan a while (and several requests) to come back from recess on time. But now his job required him to come in a few moments earlier than his peers rather than remaining outside beyond the recess period.

As Ethan's case makes clear, children have an inborn desire to help others. Similar to Ethan's door holder position, children like Anika, Liam, and Maya frequently ask their parents if they can help with simple tasks like cooking, sweeping, or mowing the lawn. These moments reflect fundamental drives that children have: a desire to master various skills and an inherent wish to make a positive difference in the lives of those around them.

But while young children exhibit this willingness to help, many parents observe that by the time they reach middle childhood, their children have seemingly grown more self-centered and sometimes want a reward for being helpful. However, parents also report that their children—while balking at helping at home—appear very willing to assist friends and teachers at school. Although the recipients of their assistance may change, the underlying desire to support others remains. This altruism requires nurturing to be transformed into a lasting sense of responsibility, compassion, and social conscience. Shaping this inherent trait is critical for both individual development and the well-being of society.

In this chapter, we'll explore various strategies for nurturing responsibility and compassion in children, examine the obstacles that parents and educators may encounter in doing so, and discuss approaches to overcoming these challenges. This chapter will offer a comprehensive guide for fostering responsibility, compassion, and social conscience in young children by focusing on the stories of Anika, Liam, and Maya.

> Our daughter experienced nausea and headaches on the Matthews Protocol, a common side effect of oxcarbazepine, especially when titrating up on the dose. I learned in the support group, that 100 mg of niacinamide (vitamin B3) given with her morning and evening dose of medication helps this temporary side effect, and it did. Also, extra hydration and electrolytes were particularly important for her in helping prevent nausea and headaches. To help alleviate her headaches, we would put a heating pad on her feet and a cold pack on her head, a common home remedy that my husband read about. I also learned that some anti-seizure medications can decrease sodium levels and oxcarbazepine is one of them. This was a concern for us because our daughter plays competitive soccer and we knew that intense, prolonged exercise can deplete sodium levels in general. Electrolytes are key in maintaining proper sodium levels on oxcarbazepine and even more so for our daughter with her intense level of training.

Nurturing Responsibility Through Positive Engagement

The evolution of qualities such as responsibility, helpfulness, and the desire to contribute can be traced back to humanity's earliest survival needs—in ancient societies, cooperation and mutual support were crucial for survival. Communities thrived by sharing resources, protecting one another, and ensuring that tasks were divided and completed. These cooperative behaviors were passed down through generations as social norms, reinforcing the value of responsibility from a young age.

As they grew up in these early societies, children learned the importance of contributing to the group's well-being. This developed into an evolutionary advantage, as those who understood this responsibility and helped ensure the survival of their communities were more likely to succeed and have offspring. Over time, these traits became deeply ingrained in human nature, making them essential for the continued growth and stability of societies.

If these qualities of responsibility and helpfulness had *not* evolved, the world would be vastly different! Communities without a sense of duty or contribution would likely be unable to function cohesively. Societies that lacked responsible individuals would face constant chaos and conflict. People would need to be even more motivated to cooperate and maintain social order, and if they failed to do so, many social structures would collapse. Without role models who demonstrated responsibility, children would grow up with fewer examples of how to be responsible themselves. Future generations would likely develop into less empathic individuals who would be less willing to help others and less inclined to work toward the common good.

In order to *not* find ourselves in these dire scenarios, it's essential to provide meaningful opportunities for children to contribute—then they'll feel a greater sense of responsibility to their overall community and society. This process begins with creating an environment that values and celebrates helpful behavior. When children feel like their contributions are appreciated and significant, they're more likely to develop a solid internal sense of responsibility. In this regard, role models (including parents, grandparents, and teachers) play a pivotal role. Children learn by observing the actions and attitudes of the adults around them. When they see responsible behavior valued and modeled, they're more inclined to adopt it themselves.

For example, Anika's parents noticed early on that she enjoyed caring for her younger brother. Rather than assigning her this role as a chore or obligation, they encouraged her to take on that responsibility by emphasizing how helpful and kind she was in her efforts. Raj and Priya would say things like, "You make such a difference when you help your brother!", thus reinforcing that her actions positively impacted those around her. This approach allowed Anika to perceive herself as not being a burden but rather being an essential contributor to her family.

Positive feedback like this is crucial for fostering responsibility, as it shifts the focus from the task to the impact of the child's actions. Children begin to see that their efforts can create real, tangible benefits for others. Furthermore, by framing tasks as contributions to the family or community rather than as chores, parents help children develop a more profound sense of purpose and pride in their responsibilities. This instills an intrinsic motivation to continue helping, leading to a lasting sense of responsibility.

> When he was young, our son tended to be consumed by his own emotions and desires and acted aggressively towards other children. It was not uncommon for other children to call him a bully, even though we felt it was rarely his intent to hurt his peers. To counter this, we've tried teaching him to notice the world around him for opportunities to help people. If a child seemed sad and had no one to sit with at lunch, we would encourage him to invite them to join him at the lunch table. When we notice people who might be less fortunate than us, we discuss ways we could help them or brighten their day. When our son tells us stories about a situation at school, we ask him how he thinks the other child in the situation feels. We continue encouraging a caring attitude by asking him if he helped or complimented anyone at school that day.

Creating a Rewarding Framework for Contribution

Intrinsic and extrinsic rewards are vital in structured environments like schools and workplaces and in personal settings such as family and friendships. These rewards help shape behaviors, reinforce values, and strengthen social bonds. Parents often use intrinsic and extrinsic rewards to encourage children to contribute to household responsibilities in family settings. For example, a child may be asked to help set the dinner table, and an extrinsic reward might be verbal praise or a small treat afterward. Over time, the child is likely to develop an intrinsic sense of satisfaction from knowing that their help is essential to the smooth functioning of family life. As they see the positive impact of their efforts on their family's daily routines, they take pride in being responsible and contributing to the household without expecting immediate external recognition. However, a positive acknowledgment by a parent—even if it's just simply saying "thank you"—is always valuable in reinforcing intrinsic motivation.

Similarly, intrinsic and extrinsic rewards play a role in deepening friendships. Friends often support each other in small but meaningful ways, such as listening, offering advice, or assisting with a task. While the initial motivation might be the appreciation and thanks that are received (extrinsic rewards), these acts of kindness foster a sense of mutual trust, loyalty, and connection (intrinsic rewards) over time. For instance, a friend who offers emotional support during tough times might feel rewarded simply by knowing that they've helped, thus developing a more profound sense of fulfillment from maintaining a solid, supportive friendship.

In family and friendship settings, the balance of intrinsic and extrinsic rewards can nurture more meaningful and sustained contributions. When people feel appreciated and recognized (extrinsic rewards), they're often more willing to invest time and effort in their relationships. Simultaneously, when they derive personal satisfaction and pride from their actions (intrinsic rewards), their commitment to helping others becomes more deeply ingrained, fostering a culture of mutual support, trust, and connection.

The importance of intrinsic and extrinsic rewards applies to every environment a child experiences: school, home, and friendships outside the classroom. As children's contributions are recognized and valued, they're more motivated to continue contributing and they develop a greater sense of responsibility, not only because of the external acknowledgments they're receiving but also because of the internal gratification that comes from knowing that their actions make a difference.

Much like Ethan's school did, Liam's school embraced a similar strategy to foster responsibility in students. In first grade, his teacher assigned him the daily task of being the class helper, a position Liam took great pride in. This role allowed him to contribute to the smooth running of the classroom by handling tasks such as distributing supplies, cleaning up, and helping other students with problems. These simple but meaningful tasks helped Liam feel like his actions were essential for the well-being of his classmates. As Liam consistently received praise and appreciation from his peers and teacher, he began to understand that his contributions were valued. This acknowledgment gave him a sense of ownership over his responsibilities and a sense of competence that extended beyond the classroom.

This early experience of being a class helper also taught Liam the significance of taking the initiative and being dependable, both of which are crucial to developing a lasting sense of responsibility. By learning that others relied on him, Liam began to see the broader impact of his actions, and that realization strengthened his motivation to continue being helpful and dependable. Such experiences in school can have a ripple effect and promote responsibility in other areas of a child's life, including in their home and social environments.

Similarly, Maya was always eager to help her mother with cooking, and she received recognition for her culinary skills. Her mother frequently invited her to assist in the kitchen, not because she needed help but because she wanted Maya to feel included in a valuable family activity. Elena consistently praised her contributions, reinforcing that helping out in the kitchen wasn't just a chore but an opportunity for Maya to develop new skills and take pride in her work. Over time, Maya's confidence in her ability grew, as did her understanding of the importance of taking on responsibilities within the family.

By encouraging children to appreciate that their efforts are meaningful at home and in school, adults reinforce a sense of responsibility that's grounded in pride, ownership, and internal motivation. This foundation is critical for cultivating responsible behavior that will last into adulthood.

> Our son has experienced how good it feels to help others in need from our yearly volunteering around Christmastime. In addition, throughout the year, we find ways to help those in need (i.e., shovel our neighbor's steps after it snows, grocery shop for a sick neighbor, hand out items to people experiencing homelessness, etc.). I am happy that our family's participation in such deeds has impacted our son's initiative to help others. He recently considered making dinner for a local business owner because her dog had been sick. He inquired if the owner's family had any food allergies, selected a recipe, and, with assistance, made the dinner and delivered it. I was proud to see his compassion for others and that he thought of this independently and followed his idea.

Encouraging Consistent Reflection on Contributions

An additional strategy for fostering responsibility is helping children reflect on the impacts of their contributions. Reflection encourages children to think about the broader contexts of their actions, helping them see that their efforts, no matter how small, have meaningful consequences. This practice cultivates a deeper understanding of responsibility beyond simply completing tasks. For example, parents can ask reflective questions such as "How do you think your help made a difference today?" or "What did you learn from helping your sibling with their homework?" These questions allow children to consider the immediate results of their actions and how those actions contribute to the well-being of others and their environment. Through this reflection, children can connect their efforts with positive outcomes. This bolsters their internal motivation and encourages them to continue contributing in the future, not for rewards but because they see the inherent value in their actions.

Additionally, these reflective practices help children build critical-thinking and problemsolving skills as they analyze how their behaviors impact the world around them. By understanding the broader implications of their actions, children can develop a more profound sense of responsibility through realizing that their contributions are essential to their immediate family *and* the larger community.

Another approach to fostering responsibility involves setting specific, achievable goals for children to work toward. These goals should be collaborative, allowing children to have input and feel empowered. For instance, when Anika resisted helping with household chores, her parents decided to involve her in creating a weekly schedule. They asked which tasks she felt most confident doing and allowed her to track her progress over time. This kind of involvement gives children a sense of control and ownership over their responsibilities—setting clear expectations and involving children in decision-making makes them more likely to feel accountable for completing their tasks.

Taking a collaborate approach to setting goals teaches valuable life skills such as time management, organization, and follow-through. As children meet their goals and witness their progress, they build confidence in their ability to handle responsibilities, thereby cultivating a sense of pride and self-reliance. Over time, these positive experiences can reinforce the idea that responsibility is not only necessary but also rewarding and fulfilling.

The Power of Compassion in Developing a Social Conscience

Emotional dysregulation—a core characteristic of children with DMDD—severely impedes children's ability to develop a social conscience. Such regulation is essential for understanding and responding to the emotions of others, which in turn forms the basis of empathy and compassion. When a child struggles with frequent and intense mood swings, irritability, and anger, their capacity to recognize and process other people's feelings is diminished. This emotional turbulence creates a barrier to learning how to empathize with others, as these children are often consumed by their own emotional distress. As a result, they may find it challenging to pause, reflect, and consider the impacts of their actions on those around them.

Furthermore, children with DMDD often experience difficulty in social interactions because their volatile emotions can lead to conflicts and strained relationships. Without the ability to effectively manage their feelings, they're less likely to engage in positive, reciprocal social exchanges that help foster a sense of community and shared responsibility. Their outbursts or mood swings may alienate peers, limiting opportunities to practice pro-social behaviors like kindness, cooperation, and understanding. Over time, this can hinder the development of a social conscience, as children who struggle with regulating their emotions cannot consistently participate in the kinds of relational dynamics that encourage empathy and moral reflection.

That said, compassion can be encouraged in all children, including children with DMDD. Anika, for instance, was naturally empathic toward others—she often noticed when her classmates felt sad or lonely and would offer a comforting word or a smile. Her teacher recognized Anika's sensitivity to others and assigned her the task of helping new students feel welcome. By giving Anika this responsibility, her teacher helped her see that small acts of kindness could significantly impact others. This experience reinforced Anika's empathy and taught her that helping others can foster a sense of belonging and community. Such experiences of empathy help children understand the ripple effects of their actions, showing them that a simple act of kindness can profoundly influence someone's day or overall well-being.

Liam, on the other hand, developed compassion through his experiences in a community service project—at age nine, he volunteered along with his family to distribute food at a local shelter. The experience left a lasting impression on him as he interacted with people facing challenging life circumstances. His parents used the opportunity to discuss the importance of helping less fortunate individuals and why acts of service are essential for a healthy community. This conversation deepened Liam's understanding of empathy and his role in the community. He began to recognize that his actions, no matter how small, could make a difference in the lives of others. Through this hands-on experience, Liam learned that empathy goes beyond feeling sympathy or feeling sorry for someone—it involves taking action to alleviate the struggles of others and promote a more equitable society.

Broadening Compassion Through Exposure to Diverse Experiences

Parents and educators can expose children to various situations and perspectives to further develop their compassion. Volunteering for a community project or at a shelter is a powerful way to nurture empathy, and sharing stories about people from different cultures, communities, or circumstances helps children understand diversity and the challenges others face. Reading books or watching films that focus on overcoming adversity, caring for others, or addressing social injustices can also spark essential conversations.

In Maya's case, her journey toward compassion took a different path. Not surprisingly, as a young child, Maya was primarily concerned with her needs and desires the way most children are. However, when her parents adopted a stray dog from a shelter, Maya was responsible for caring for the dog. This new responsibility required her to consider the needs of another living being, a role that significantly expanded her capacity for empathy. Over time, Maya's understanding of compassion deepened as she realized that caring for others—whether people or animals—requires dedication and selflessness.

Modeling Compassionate Behavior

One of the most effective ways to instill compassion in children is through modeling it. Children are keen observers of the world around them and often learn more from what they see than from what they're told. When they witness parents, teachers, or caregivers treating others with kindness, offering help to those in need, or standing up against injustice, they internalize these behaviors and view them as ordinary and necessary parts of life. Modeling compassion in everyday interactions provides children with real-world examples of being considerate, empathic, and socially responsible.

For example, if a parent regularly helps a neighbor by carrying groceries or offering a listening ear during tough times, children are likely to notice these actions and begin to understand the importance of lending a hand to others. These acts may seem small, but they can significantly impact a child's development of empathy. Children who see kindness in action will be more likely to replicate it at home and in broader social settings, such as in school or within their greater community.

Parents can also actively involve children in simple acts of kindness, making the practice of compassion a shared family activity. For instance, a family might gather gently used clothes or toys that are no longer needed and donate them to a local shelter. Engaging children in conversations about the importance of giving to others who are less fortunate helps them connect their actions to the needs of the community. Similarly, writing cards or drawing pictures for elderly neighbors or nursing home residents can teach children that small gestures of thoughtfulness can have a profound impact on someone's day.

Community involvement is yet another powerful way to teach children compassion. Families can participate in neighborhood clean-ups, food drives, or charity events, where children see firsthand how helping others contributes to the greater good. In these settings, children are exposed to different perspectives and challenges that people may face, which broadens their understanding of the world and nurtures a more profound sense of empathy. Participating in a food drive might prompt a child to ask why people are hungry, for example, opening up a valuable conversation about inequality and how acts of service can help address such issues.

Moreover, when adults model standing up against injustice, they teach children that compassion also involves defending the rights and dignity of others. This could include supporting a friend being bullied at school, participating in a peaceful protest for a cause, or speaking out against harmful behavior. Children learn that compassion is about kindness in individual acts and contributing to a fair and equitable society.

Overcoming Obstacles in Teaching Responsibility and Compassion

While nurturing responsibility and compassion in children is rewarding, it has challenges. Children, like adults, are only sometimes motivated to contribute, especially when the tasks assigned to them feel mundane or repetitive. Moreover, developmental stages can bring about natural phases of resistance as children assert their independence and test boundaries.

Anika, for example, went through a phase where she resisted helping her parents around the house. After several reminders to complete her chores, she would respond with excuses or simply avoid the tasks altogether. This behavior left her parents feeling frustrated and uncertain about how to encourage responsibility without resorting to constant nagging. To address this, they reframed chores as opportunities for her to take ownership. Instead of saying, "You need to clean your room," they asked, "How can we help you make your room feel like your own space?" This subtle shift in language made Anika feel more in control of the task, allowing her to approach it with a greater sense of responsibility.

Liam also experienced obstacles in developing responsibility, particularly when it came to keeping up with his schoolwork—as a naturally active child, he struggled to sit still and complete his homework. His parents tried different strategies to help him focus, but nothing worked. Finally, his teacher introduced a reward system where Liam could earn extra playtime by completing his assignments. Although this method was influential in the short term, Liam's parents were concerned that he was becoming too reliant on external rewards. To address this, they gradually shifted the focus from external rewards to internal satisfaction—they began to praise Liam for his effort and hard work, helping him see that the real reward came from doing his best. Over time, Liam developed a stronger sense of responsibility for his schoolwork, motivated by pride in his accomplishments rather than the promise of a reward.

For her part, Maya displayed frustration when it became challenging to take care of her dog. Initially excited about the responsibility, Maya soon realized that feeding, walking, and grooming the dog required daily efforts, and she began to neglect some of her duties. That led her parents to step in, although instead of punishing her or taking over the responsibilities, they sat down with her to discuss the importance of caring for another living being. They encouraged her to create a schedule for the dog's care, giving her more control over the tasks. This approach helped Maya develop a sense of ownership and pride in her responsibilities, ultimately fostering a more profound commitment to the well-being of her pet.

Implementing Collaborative Problem-Solving

Engaging children in collaborative problem-solving is a powerful way to overcome obstacles. Rather than dictating solutions, parents can work with children to identify the root causes of resistance and brainstorm strategies to overcome them. This method addresses the immediate issue and also teaches children essential life skills such as critical thinking, negotiation, and perseverance. Collaborative problem-solving fosters a sense of autonomy by giving children a voice in decision-making and reinforcing the belief that challenges can be overcome with creativity and effort.

Anika consistently resisted cleaning her room. Instead of imposing consequences or doing the task for her, however, her parents took a collaborative approach: they sat down with Anika and asked her to explain why cleaning her room was difficult or unappealing. Anika explained that the task felt overwhelming because too many toys and clothes were scattered around. Together, she and her parents brainstormed solutions. One of Anika's suggestions was to break the task into smaller steps, such as focusing on one area of the room at a time. Raj and Priya agreed and decided to make the process more fun by setting a timer to see how quickly she could tidy each section. This collaborative approach solved the immediate problem and simultaneously empowered Anika to take ownership of her space and manage her responsibilities in a way that worked for her.

Similarly, Liam needed help with completing his homework on time. Instead of punishing him for unfinished assignments, his parents worked with him to identify the underlying issues. Liam explained that he had difficulty concentrating after school because he was too tired and distracted. Liam, his parents, and his teacher collaboratively discussed ways to improve his focus. They all decided that Liam could start his homework after having a snack and a short break, during which time he could engage in physical activity to release his pent-up energy. They also created a structured homework routine with frequent breaks. During this collaborative problem-solving session, Liam was encouraged to offer his input, an invitation that helped him feel more in control of his study habits. It also gave him a practical solution that addressed his needs without him feeling external pressures.

Maya resisted feeding her dog because she found the task to be repetitive and she sometimes forgot about it altogether. But her parents didn't scold her—instead, they asked her why she struggled with her responsibility. Maya admitted that she often forgot and didn't feel motivated to feed the dog daily. David and Elena suggested they work together to create a feeding schedule, and Maya proposed making a fun chart that she could put stickers on each time she completed a task. This collaborative approach addressed Maya's resistance and helped her feel more engaged with and responsible for her pet's care.

In these examples, taking a collaborative approach allowed the children to participate in problem-solving, making them feel more invested in the outcome. It also shifted the dynamic from a parent-child power struggle to a cooperative effort wherein both sides worked toward a mutually beneficial solution. This method fosters resilience, self-confidence, and a sense of shared responsibility and shows children that challenges can be managed and overcome with creativity and teamwork.

Teaching Self-Regulation and Emotional Management

Another significant challenge arises when dealing with children diagnosed with DMDD, namely that they struggle to manage their emotions. These children often struggle with extreme irritability and frequent temper outbursts disproportionate to the situation, and as a result, managing their emotions during overwhelming or frustrating tasks can be particularly difficult. The emotional volatility associated with DMDD makes it tough for these children to develop self-regulation skills, which cascades into lessening their ability to demonstrate compassion and empathy. Parents and caregivers must be patient and consistent in helping these children manage their emotions. Teaching self-regulation requires a structured approach that incorporates frequent emotional check-ins, coping mechanisms, and clear boundaries. Validating children's emotional experiences while guiding them through calming strategies is crucial. Over time, with support, children with DMDD can begin to manage their emotions more effectively, leading to improved emotional resilience and an improved ability to engage in tasks.

For instance, Maya became frustrated when her math homework seemed too complicated. Instead of simply telling her to keep trying, David and Elena took the time to help her identify and express her frustration. They encouraged her to say, "I'm feeling frustrated because this is hard for me," helping Maya understand that it was okay to feel that way. They then introduced simple techniques like deep breathing exercises to help her manage her emotions, and they also created a "calm-down corner," a quiet space where Maya could take a few minutes to relax and regain her focus whenever she felt overwhelmed. Once Maya had calmed down, she was able to approach the math problem with more clarity. This process taught Maya to better handle frustration, and it also reinforced her ability to work through complex tasks.

Parents can help their children manage their emotions and refocus on their responsibilities by teaching them self-regulation techniques like mindfulness and by creating calming spaces; all of these tactics can foster a more resilient and self-compassionate approach to challenges. Many children with DMDD struggle to express what exactly is frustrating them so that someone else can help them resolve the issue and continue to complete their work. (When these children become overwhelmed, they have a tendency to shut down and say they "can't" finish the task at hand.) After they cool down, it's important that parents guide them to return to work and help them get over whatever speed bump/issue they've gotten stuck on. This guidance shows children how to see the small steps within a larger assignment, making it seem less overwhelming.

Conclusion: The Path to Responsibility, Compassion, and Social Conscience

Helping children develop a sense of responsibility, compassion, and social conscience is a multifaceted process that requires patience, understanding, and guidance. Parents, grandparents, and educators can cultivate these essential qualities by nurturing children's innate desire to help and by providing them with meaningful opportunities to contribute. When caregivers foster a sense of responsibility early on, children learn the value of being accountable for their actions and decisions, making it easier for them to grow into conscientious individuals.

When parents approach the challenges in their child's life with empathy and a collaborative spirit, they can guide their children toward becoming responsible, compassionate individuals aware of their roles in creating a just and caring society. This ongoing process requires parents and other caregivers to consistently reinforce moral values and model empathic behaviors. As children grow up, these lessons about responsibility, compassion, and social conscience will continue to shape their actions and decisions, empowering them to become change makers in their communities and beyond.

Chapter 12
Establishing a Partnership with Your Child's School

Emma's Story

Emma Rodriguez, a bright and creative seven-year-old, was diagnosed with DMDD shortly after she started first grade. Her parents Jose and Maria had noticed that unlike other children her age, Emma's moods could shift quickly and intensely. "What started as minor frustrations would often escalate into explosive outbursts," said Maria. Jose added, "We noticed that Emma's ability to manage these intense feelings was limited." These episodes were frequent at home, and when Emma entered school, her challenges grew more apparent, especially when she was in a structured environment with new demands and increased peer interactions.

Emma's teachers were quick to notice her difficulties in the classroom. She often struggled with transitions, such as moving from one activity to the next, and she became overwhelmed by simple frustrations, like not being able to immediately grasp a math concept or if her group didn't follow her suggestions during collaborative activities. While many children have occasional emotional outbursts, Emma's outbursts were more intense and frequent. "We would get almost daily calls from school telling us that Emma was crying uncontrollably, yelling, or even throwing things when her emotions became too overwhelming," reported Maria.

The noise and unpredictability of the classroom also seemed to amplify Emma's emotional dysregulation. Situations that other children could brush off—a misplaced backpack, a change in the schedule—could lead to hours of distress for Emma. Her peers, although kind, did not understand her reactions, and that made it challenging for Emma to form friendships. Her academic performance also began to suffer because her emotional struggles were consuming so much of her energy and focus.

After Emma was diagnosed with DMDD, her parents sought the help of a child psychiatrist and a therapist who specialized in emotional regulation for young children. Emma's treatment plan included a combination of cognitive-behavioral therapy (CBT) to help her develop coping skills for managing her intense emotions and family therapy to improve communication and understanding at home. Emma also participated in social skills training sessions, where she learned how to navigate peer relationships and respond to social challenges in a more measured way. Although medication wasn't immediately prescribed, her doctor closely monitored her progress, and after several months of therapy, Emma's care team added the combination of medications used in the Matthews Protocol to help stabilize Emma's mood swings. The combination of therapy, medication, and continued emotional support from her parents created a comprehensive treatment plan, giving Emma the tools to better manage her emotions both at home and at school.

Aware of her diagnosis and struggles, Jose and Maria realized that without support at school, Emma might continue to fall behind both socially and academically. They reached out to the school to set up a meeting, hoping to develop a plan that would address Emma's unique needs in the classroom.

At the meeting, they discussed Emma's behavior with her teacher, the school psychologist, and the principal. Emma's teacher shared her observations: while Emma was intelligent and had much potential, her emotional responses were interfering with her ability to succeed in class. The school psychologist, familiar with DMDD, explained to the team how children like Emma can struggle with emotional regulation, especially in the face of frustration or change.

With the input of the school psychologist and Emma's teacher, they all jointly developed an Individualized Education Plan (IEP) to create a supportive environment for Emma at school. This plan included several key components, including the following:

Emotional Regulation Strategies

The school counselor worked with Emma on techniques to manage her emotions, such as taking deep breaths, using sensory tools (like a stress ball), and identifying when she was beginning to feel overwhelmed. They created a "calm-down corner" in the classroom where Emma could go when she felt her emotions building up. This space was also available to other students so that Emma didn't feel singled out. However, it was primarily occupied by Emma.

Structured Routines

Since Emma struggled with transitions, her teacher began providing her with a visual schedule so she could see what was coming next. The teacher also gave Emma advance notice of any changes in the routine, which helped reduce her anxiety.

Positive Reinforcement

Emma thrived on encouragement, so her teacher used positive reinforcement (primarily in the form of verbal praise) to acknowledge moments when Emma was able to regulate her emotions. Even small successes like asking for help instead of getting upset were complimented, feedback that made Emma feel more in control and capable.

Frequent Check-Ins

The school counselor scheduled regular check-ins with Emma to ensure that she was feeling supported and to help her process any challenges from the day.

Parent Involvement

Emma's parents stayed closely involved, attending bimonthly meetings with the teacher to monitor Emma's progress. They worked with Emma at home on the same emotional regulation strategies she was learning at school, ensuring consistency between her home and school environments.

Within a few months, Emma's behavior at school began to improve. She still had difficult days, but they were becoming less frequent. With the support of her teacher and the strategies she was learning, Emma was gaining confidence in her ability to manage her emotions. She started to feel more comfortable in group activities and even began making friends. The calm-down corner became a place where she could take a break before her feelings escalated. Her academic performance also improved as she spent more time focusing on her work and less time feeling overwhelmed by frustration.

The partnership between Emma's parents and the school was key to her progress—the consistent communication and collaborative problem-solving helped create a supportive and understanding environment for Emma. Her parents also felt more empowered because they knew they had a team at school who understood their daughter's needs and was invested in her success.

As Emma moved into second grade, her Behavior Intervention Plan (BIP) evolved with her needs. Her first-grade teacher shared her insights with her new teacher, ensuring a smooth transition. The school staff and her parents continued to monitor Emma's progress, adjusting her behavior plan and accommodations as needed.

Emma's story highlights the importance of a strong parent-school partnership when it comes to supporting children with DMDD. Through collaboration, patience, and understanding, Emma was able to overcome many of her challenges at school, setting herself on a path toward continued growth and success.

Building a strong partnership with a child's school isn't merely advantageous, it's essential for their academic achievement and personal growth, especially when managing conditions like DMDD. Solid relationships between parents and schools that are grounded in open communication, trust, and mutual respect mean that both parties will align their goals to provide children with optimal educational and emotional support. This collaboration is even more critical when a child faces behavioral or emotional challenges that may impact their school experience. As educational practices continue to evolve given the integration of more and more technology, changing curriculum standards, and a growing focus on mental health, parents and schools must cooperate even more closely.

Taking a proactive approach to parent-school partnerships helps create a consistent and supportive framework that enhances the child's growth. Ideally, this partnership starts from the very first interaction with the school and extends throughout the child's educational journey. In this chapter, we will explore strategies, principles, and practices that parents—especially those of children with DMDD—can adopt to build and maintain a positive and productive relationship with their child's school. This partnership is not only vital for improving academic performance but is also essential for the child's emotional and social well-being. Interventions with Maya, Liam, Anika, and their parents will illustrate how these principles can be applied in real-life situations to ensure a child's success in school despite the challenges posed by DMDD.

Many parents are unaware of their children's educational rights under the Individuals with Disabilities Education Improvement Act (IDEIA) and Section 504 of the Americans with Disabilities Act (ADA). These laws ensure that students with disabilities such as DMDD receive the support they need to succeed in school. However, many families mistakenly believe that from the outset, they must choose *between* an IEP (under IDEIA) and a 504 plan. They do not. But parents do need to understand that the first step should be a thorough assessment of their child's needs.

Such an assessment focuses on identifying the accommodations, services, or specialized instruction necessary for the child to access and benefit from their education in the least restrictive environment. Rather than predetermining a specific support plan, parents and schools should collaborate to determine which interventions are essential for the child's success. For a brief, comprehensive guide to understanding these laws and processes, parents can refer to Appendix B at the end of this book—there, we outline critical rights, eligibility criteria, and procedural safeguards under both IDEIA and Section 504. Once parents are empowered with this knowledge, they can advocate effectively for their child's education and seek support that's tailored precisely to their child's needs.

How the Brain Learns

One of the most challenging therapeutic tasks has been to explain to parents, educational and medical professionals, and even children how the brain and mind work. In the past, for example, when a child struggled to learn to read, many parents were told that their child suffered from a reading disorder. When parents asked what had led to this conclusion, they often heard a rather simplistic response: "Because your child is struggling to read." Fortunately, over the past several decades, the science of neuropsychology has begun to provide more sophisticated answers to this and other developmental challenges that children face. With this knowledge, more effective teaching and therapy strategies are being developed.

After thousands of evaluations, specialists have come to understand and appreciate the differences between the developing brain and the mind, as well as the differences between ability, knowledge, and skill. When parents bring their child in for an initial evaluation, these differences are one of the first things that should be discussed. Though a diagnosis is still valuable, it's no longer a sufficient explanation of the problem.

The goal of an assessment is not to add up behaviors and proclaim diagnoses but rather to assist parents, educators, physicians, and other adults in the child's life to see the world through the eyes of the child. To accomplish this goal, parents must understand that an initial view of their child's developing brain focuses on three phenomena:

Ability

Abilities are the genetically driven, biological qualities that all of us bring to the world. These qualities are not evenly distributed among people—some of us are more advanced in certain abilities and some of us are weaker in certain abilities. These include not only physical abilities (e.g., balance and coordination) but also cognitive abilities (memory, reasoning, thinking, attention, planning, sequencing, etc.). Abilities are in fact hardwired. But that should not be interpreted as saying that children cannot be assisted to strengthen their less-developed abilities and be successful in life! Knowing that abilities are hardwired is simply knowing that children may not attain the same level of proficiency in certain abilities as their peers will. However, they can still be successful if parents and professionals are sufficiently enlightened about their individual strengths and weaknesses. It's equally important to identify and build on a child's naturally strong abilities.

Knowledge

Knowledge is everything we learn through our experiences. While that includes our academic experiences, knowledge goes far beyond scholarly endeavors. For example, language is knowledge—if we don't speak to children, they'll never learn to speak. Socialization, too, is dependent on knowledge. A child may have all the genetics they need to socialize appropriately, but if they're never given the opportunity to interact with other children or adults, they won't know how to do so.

Our abilities help us acquire knowledge. For some children, this may be an accelerated process; for others, slow is fast enough. Parents can be taught to change their minds and adjust their expectations to accept and even embrace the pace their child will need to adhere to in order to acquire knowledge, emotional regulation, self-discipline, and social skills.

Skill

Abilities are used to acquire knowledge, but simply possessing knowledge and ability is just the foundation—we must actually *use* our knowledge and ability to solve problems in all areas of our lives. Taking this perspective, skill is not a noun (e.g., a reading skill) but a verb (e.g., skillfully reading). All kinds of factors can impair skill. Some children may possess excellent coordination and be very good athletes, yet are not skillful in competition because they're nervous, impulsive, or ill-prepared. Other children may have an average ability to sequence and associate and be average readers but be very successful in school because they're skillful at meeting all of their responsibilities.

Appreciating these developmental phenomena—ability, knowledge, and skill—provides parents with a firm, reasoned, and reasonable basis that allows them to better understand their children and themselves.

The Unique Challenges of DMDD in School

Children with DMDD face a range of unique and complex challenges in the school environment that affect both their emotional well-being and their academic performance. Emotionally, these children may struggle to form and maintain stable peer relationships due to their unpredictable and intense emotional outbursts. Such behavior can lead to misunderstandings and alienation from classmates, which in turn often causes feelings of rejection and isolation. This social isolation exacerbates their emotional volatility, creating a harmful cycle where frustration and anger build up, leading to more frequent outbursts. The heightened emotional state that children with DMDD experience can also make it difficult for them to concentrate on academic tasks, further impeding their learning and overall school performance. In short, emotional and academic struggles can overwhelm the child and make school a particularly stressful environment.

Teachers and school staff also face challenges when managing students with DMDD. Their unpredictable behavior can disrupt the classroom and make it difficult to maintain order and meet the needs of other students, for example. In many cases, the disciplinary actions that may be taken in response to such emotional outbursts are punitive and counterproductive. They often fail to address the root causes of the behavior (i.e., emotional dysregulation) and spark a series of repeated incidents and strained relationships between the child and their educators. To avoid these unfortunate situations, all school personnel must become increasingly knowledgeable about DMDD, how this disorder might manifest in the school environment, and which effective interventions can be implemented.

The Role of Parents in the Educational Process

Parents play an integral role in their child's educational journey, especially when that child has DMDD. Parents are often the first ones to notice signs of emotional dysregulation and can provide invaluable insights into their child's needs and triggers. By working closely with teachers, school counselors, and administrators, parents can ensure that their child receives the appropriate accommodations and support in the school environment.

When a child is struggling with DMDD and parents and teachers are at a loss as to how to best to help that child, these significant adults in the child's life must avoid blaming each other. Instead, they must acknowledge the challenges of raising and teaching a child with DMDD and then collaborate on implementing effective strategies to help the child succeed at home and at school.

Maya's story illustrates the importance of parents and school staff working closely together. Her parents noticed early on that she became easily overwhelmed in noisy, unstructured environments. At school, this meant that transitions between classes and activities often led to explosive emotional outbursts. By collaborating with her teacher, Maya's parents were able to develop a plan that helped Maya transition more smoothly. This included giving her extra time to move from one activity to another and allowing her to use noise-canceling headphones in particularly loud settings. Since loud noise could easily be a trigger for Maya, her parents requested that her IEP include that she receive advance notice before a fire drill so she could be prepared with her noise-canceling headphones ahead of time. This kind of collaboration helped Maya feel more in control, reducing the frequency of her outbursts and allowing her to focus more on her schoolwork.

In situations like Maya's, parental involvement goes beyond attending school events or helping with homework. It requires a commitment to showing the child that learning is a shared endeavor and that their parents are working with their school to support them. For children with DMDD, this might mean communicating frequently with the school about emotional triggers, jointly helping to develop behavior management strategies, and reinforcing these strategies at home. When parents are involved in this way, they help create a seamless, supportive experience for their child across both their home and school environments.

Expanding Parent Involvement: The Broader Impact

For children like 10-year-old Liam, parental involvement is about more than monitoring homework or participating in school events. Liam was experiencing frequent mood swings that sometimes resulted in disruptive behavior during class. His parents were deeply involved in his education, and they noticed that his frustration often stemmed from academic struggles, particularly when it came to math. By actively engaging with his teacher and the school counselor, Liam's parents helped develop a tailored support plan that included him having a quiet space where he could retreat when he felt overwhelmed. They also worked with his teacher to adjust his workload and allow him extra time to complete difficult assignments. On days that were particularly difficult for Liam, his teacher reduced the number of math problems that he was required to complete.

> Within weeks of starting kindergarten, my son couldn't keep his hands off other students and would threaten harm to teachers. In the first grade, he got mad at recess, hit a teacher, and tried to run away from school. With a new diagnosis of DMDD and a 504 Plan, his teachers had solid ideas for smoother transitions between activities. They gave him breaks from the classroom, provided scheduled check-ins with a trusted counselor, and enrolled him in social skills classes throughout the school. It helped for a while, but as soon as the novelty wore off, the old behaviors quickly returned. After a formal evaluation, my son qualified for an IEP, which provided our son with specific goals and access to a paraprofessional aid that would help him process things if needed. He had morning check-ins to prevent irritability from escalating. The school even matched him to mentor an autistic child, which helped him learn empathy and focus on someone other than himself. He later tested into the academically and intellectually gifted program and was challenged with books and conversations that stimulated him.

Parental involvement in this case included advocating for Liam's emotional needs while also helping him manage his frustration with schoolwork. By remaining actively and respectfully engaged with the school, Liam's parents provided him with the tools he needed to succeed academically while also fostering his emotional development. The broader impact of this involvement extended beyond Liam's academic achievements—it also helped him build resilience, develop coping strategies, and improve his interactions with peers and teachers.

> After my son had been on therapeutic levels of Matthews Protocol for about three months, he was still experiencing intermittent outbursts relating to certain activities as well as significant negative self-talk. We, along with our son's provider, felt that he was experiencing a significant amount of anxiety and depression that was masked by his chronic irritability in the past. The protocol improved his mood and outburst frequency but did little for his anxiety and depression. Adding additional medication to address this anxiety and depression played a huge role in his long-term stability to date. There are several DMDD children on Matthews Protocol who did not have anxiety/depression as preadolescents. The parents of these children consequently saw a dramatic increase in anxiety/depression during puberty which manifested itself as increased anger, threatening their previous stability. These parents reported that their children were able to return to stability after additional medication was added to target the new increase in anxiety/depression.

For families managing DMDD, regular participation in and communication with the school can make a significant difference in their child's success. When parents, educators, and counselors work together, they create a structured and supportive environment that allows the child to navigate their emotions more effectively, leading to better outcomes both academically and socially.

Addressing Barriers to Parental Involvement

While parent involvement is critical, it's not without its challenges. Work commitments, language barriers, and past negative experiences with schools can hinder a parent's ability to engage fully in their child's education. Anika's parents experienced this firsthand. When Anika was diagnosed with DMDD at age 11, her parents—both working full-time—struggled to find time to meet with the school to discuss accommodations. Additionally, they were unfamiliar with the school system and unsure of their rights when it came to advocating for Anika.

Anika's case underscores the importance of schools offering flexible opportunities for parental involvement. Her school helped overcome the barriers her family initially faced by scheduling virtual meetings that fit her parents' schedules and providing them with resources about her rights under the Individuals with Disabilities Education Act. As a result, Raj and Priya felt more knowledgeable about what the school was required to offer and were able to take an active role in developing Anika's IEP, ensuring that her emotional and academic needs were addressed.

Schools can make a tremendous difference by acknowledging and addressing these kinds of barriers. By offering flexible meeting times, translation services, and resources that inform parents of their rights, schools can ensure that *all* families can participate fully in their child's education regardless of their circumstances. This support is especially important for parents of children with DMDD—those parents may need additional guidance in navigating the school system and advocating for their child's needs.

The School's Role in Supporting Parental Involvement

Schools play an essential role in fostering parental involvement, particularly when a child has DMDD. Educators and administrators must recognize that conditions like DMDD require effective management strategies and consistent collaboration with parents. Schools that actively seek out ways to engage parents in their children's education often see better outcomes, as this partnership helps create a cohesive support system for the child.

Creating a welcoming and inclusive school environment is a vital step in supporting parental involvement. Schools that embrace diversity and prioritize open communication are more likely to see active participation from families. For example, Liam's school regularly hosted workshops for parents of children with special needs, offering resources and strategies for managing behavioral challenges both at home and in the classroom. These types of workshops provide a platform for parents to learn from each other as well as from school staff, leading to a greater sense of community and shared responsibility.

For children with DMDD, it's especially important that schools create clear and consistent communication channels. Maya's school, for example, implemented a daily communication log in which her teacher could note any significant emotional or behavioral challenges. This log was shared with Maya's parents, who used it to track patterns in her behavior and to reinforce positive coping strategies at home. This consistent feedback helped both the school and Maya's family stay aligned in their approach and ultimately reduced the frequency and severity of Maya's emotional outbursts.

Building Open Lines of Communication

Early and open communication between parents and teachers is crucial in managing DMDD—such communication sets the tone for a collaborative relationship that focuses on the child's needs. Liam's parents, for example, introduced themselves to his new teacher at the start of the school year, explaining his DMDD diagnosis and discussing potential triggers. This initial conversation helped the teacher anticipate and manage Liam's outbursts, preventing situations that could have led to further frustration.

Having regular check-ins between parents and teachers is equally important. Anika's parents met with her teacher once a month to review her progress and discuss any new concerns. These meetings allowed both parties to adjust strategies as needed, ensuring that Anika's academic and emotional needs were being met. The sessions also helped maintain positive connections between home and school, reinforcing a team approach to Anika's education.

When challenges arise, it's essential for parents to approach these conversations constructively. For instance, when Liam's behavior began to deteriorate during math class, his parents worked with his teacher to develop new approaches. Instead of blaming the school for his struggles, they focused on finding practical solutions like using stress-reduction techniques and giving him short breaks during challenging tasks. A collaborative approach like this fosters trust and ensures that everyone is working toward the same goal: bolstering the child's well-being.

Understanding School Policies and Procedures

For parents of children with DMDD, understanding school policies is critical to ensure that their child receives the necessary accommodations and support. Schools have guidelines that govern behavior management, disciplinary actions, and academic expectations, and parents must be familiar with these policies in order to advocate for their child effectively.

In Anika's case, her parents were initially unaware of the school's policies regarding behavioral interventions. After researching the school's guidelines and attending a parent workshop on the topic, they were better prepared to work with the school to develop an effective IEP that included accommodations for her emotional outbursts. Knowing what support the school was required to provide helped Raj and Priya ensure that Anika received the care she needed to thrive in the classroom.

Parents should also be aware of the school's administrative structure. For instance, Maya's parents found it helpful to build relationships not only with her teacher but also with the school counselor and principal. Then when Maya began experiencing more frequent mood swings, the counselor worked with her parents and teacher to implement additional coping strategies. This coordinated effort ensured that Maya received consistent support across all aspects of her school day. In addition, having regular sessions with her school counselor was an added layer of support and comfort for Maya. She developed a connection with her counselor, whom she viewed as a safe and trusted person who was available to support her during difficult days.

Supporting a Child's Learning at Home

How well a child can manage DMDD often depends on the continuity of support between home and school. Liam's parents created a quiet, structured space at home for completing homework, which helped him focus without becoming overwhelmed. They also reinforced the coping strategies he learned at school, such as using a stress ball or taking deep breaths when he felt frustrated. By maintaining consistency between home and school, Michael and Sarah helped Liam feel more secure and better equipped to handle emotional challenges.

Positive reinforcement is another key element of supporting a child's learning. Maya's parents made a point of celebrating her successes, both big and small. When she successfully navigated a difficult social interaction at school, they praised her effort and encouraged her to continue using the coping skills she had developed. This positive reinforcement helped Maya build confidence and motivated her to keep working on her emotional regulation.

Regular communication about schoolwork and behavior is also essential. In Anika's case, her parents reviewed her homework assignments and behavior reports with her every evening. This routine kept them informed about her progress and allowed Anika to reflect on her day and discuss any challenges she had faced. By consistently engaging with Anika's daily experiences, her parents provided the guidance and support she needed to succeed.

Overcoming Common Challenges in Parent-School Partnerships

Parents of children with DMDD often face a range of challenges as they begin to build a strong partnership with their children's schools. Because DMDD is characterized by severe temper outbursts and irritability, it can be difficult for educators unfamiliar with the condition to understand the child's behavior. This often leads to misinterpretations and friction between the school and the family. Understanding the nature of these challenges is crucial for developing practical solutions that foster collaboration and ensure the child's success in an academic environment.

Differences in Communication Styles

One of the primary challenges in the relationship between parents and school staff is the significant differences in communication styles. Schools tend to adopt formal and structured methods of communication, often utilizing scheduled meetings, written reports, and formal emails. This procedural approach is meant to ensure clarity, organization, and accountability.

However, for parents, this method may seem rigid and impersonal—to feel connected to their child's daily experiences, many parents prefer a more informal and ongoing dialogue with regular, casual updates. They may seek more spontaneous conversations or feedback, especially concerning their child's well-being and progress. These contrasting communication preferences can unfortunately lead to misunderstandings. Parents may feel left out or uninformed and think they're not receiving enough information about their child's development. On the other hand, schools may feel overwhelmed by parents' frequent requests for updates and perceive them as a strain on their time and resources. All of this can create tension between both parties. The challenge becomes how to bridge the gaps and find a balanced approach to communication that satisfies both sides.

Solution

To address the communication gap between schools and parents, it's essential to establish a clear, structured, and mutually agreed-upon communication plan. The plan should focus on accommodating the school's need for procedural communication and the parent's desire for ongoing dialogue. One potential solution is for schools to provide regular updates through the preferred communication channels of both parties, such as emails, phone calls, or in-person meetings. This could involve weekly or biweekly check-ins to keep parents informed about critical developments while avoiding the overload of daily updates.

Furthermore, appointing a designated point of contact at the school (perhaps a special education coordinator or a specific teacher) can ensure consistency and reliability in communication. This individual serves as the liaison between the parents and the school, providing timely updates and promptly addressing concerns. Agreeing on the method and frequency of communication will help both parties stay aligned, reduce the potential for miscommunication, and build a stronger, more cooperative relationship. Schools and parents can work together more effectively when they proactively manage communication expectations to support every child's education.

Conflicting Schedules

One of the recurring challenges in the relationship between parents and school staff is managing conflicting schedules—both parents and educators often have demanding commitments, making it difficult to find mutually convenient times to meet or discuss a child's progress. Parents may be juggling work, family responsibilities, and personal obligations, and at the same time, teachers and school staff must adhere to structured school hours and balance their commitments to multiple students. These time constraints can lead to frustration, especially when timely communication is essential to address a behavioral issue or an academic concern.

Sometimes the inability to find a convenient meeting time results in delayed discussions, further complicating matters if the child's struggles require immediate intervention. An ongoing scheduling challenge can create a disconnect between the school and the parents and leave both sides unable to effectively communicate and address the child's needs promptly.

Solution

To overcome the issue of conflicting schedules, both parties must exercise flexibility and prioritize the child's needs when arranging meetings or discussions. One way to do this is by considering alternative meeting formats like virtual sessions or phone calls when in-person meetings aren't feasible. Virtual platforms in particular can provide a convenient solution, allowing parents and school staff to connect outside of traditional working hours.

Schools can also offer written summaries or video recordings of important meetings, presentations, or events. This ensures that parents who cannot attend in person still receive the necessary information, reducing the risk of them feeling uninformed. Another option is to establish a system where short updates can be provided through email or shared documents, allowing parents to stay engaged without attending lengthy meetings. Prioritizing regular, brief communication helps keep parents in the loop without requiring frequent and time-consuming appointments. By adopting a flexible, proactive approach to communication and scheduling, schools and parents can better collaborate to support the child's progress and also ensure that meaningful conversations aren't delayed due to logistical challenges.

Misunderstanding a Child's Behavior

Misunderstanding a child's behavior, particularly when they have DMDD, is one of the most significant challenges parents face. Children with DMDD often exhibit irritability, temper outbursts, and aggressive behaviors that stem from their difficulty in regulating emotions, and unfortunately, teachers and school personnel who aren't trained in mental health issues may misinterpret these behaviors as willful defiance, disrespect, or poor discipline. For example, a child might have an outburst due to feeling overwhelming frustration, but teachers might interpret that as deliberate misbehavior. The result is often assigning punitive measures— detention, suspension, removal from the classroom—that fail to address the underlying emotional or mental health needs of the child. In fact, such disciplinary actions can exacerbate the situation by increasing the child's anxiety, frustration, and feelings of isolation. Over time, this can harm the child's emotional well-being and create tension between the parents and the school. (That's exactly what happened with Anika—her outbursts were misinterpreted as defiance.) This kind of lack of understanding affects the child and can damage the trust between parents and educators, making it harder for both parties to work together to support the child's needs.

The importance of teachers becoming knowledgeable about DMDD and not misinterpreting a child's behavior was captured by the different perceptions that two teachers had of Sonya, a moody eight-year-old girl with a history of explosive episodes. Her third-grade teacher reported that Sonya could have excellent days at school, defining "excellent" as "behaving appropriately, following rules, and completing her work." In contrast, on other days, Sonya would blurt out answers, yell at a peer, or go to the bathroom without asking permission.

Sonya's seemingly inconsistent behaviors from one day to the next led her teacher to conclude, "Sonya could do the work and behave appropriately if she wanted to, but it seems that on certain days she has decided not to do so. I'm not certain why she's made that decision, but she has to learn not to misbehave!"

In an initial meeting with a therapist, when the therapist asked Sonya's parents about Sonya's islands of competence, they reported that she loved to read and that while she could be a "handful" for them as parents, younger children gravitated toward her and enjoyed having her read stories to them. Sonya's mother observed, "You would think she was a different child when she's reading to a couple of six-year-old neighbors! She looks so happy and is so patient with them. Sonya loves the school librarian! If she were allowed, she would spend all day in the library."

Given her interests and strengths, Sonya's therapist suggested a couple of school interventions. One involved having Sonya assist in the library for an hour a week; the other included having her read to several kindergarteners and first-grade students for an hour or two a week.

Sonya's teacher resisted these recommendations, contending, "We should not be reinforcing negative behavior." Her opinion of Sonya didn't change—she staunchly believed that Sonya could control her behavior if she wanted to and that she would have to "earn" the privilege of assisting in the library.

Fortunately, only a few more weeks remained in the school year. When school resumed in the fall, Sonya's fourth-grade teacher understood that Sonya couldn't control her behavior. Her fourth-grade teacher believed in a strength-based approach and decided that Sonya's program would immediately include assisting the school librarian and reading to younger children. With this empathic, compassionate teacher supporting her and thanks to the time she was allowed to spend helping in the library and reading to younger children, Sonya's behavior improved significantly in school. Her parents reported that Sonya made gains at home, too, as they likewise learned to focus more on her strengths and interests.

> When our daughter was 10 years old, and in the 5th grade, she had a 504 plan in place that was not preventing continued disruptions to the classroom and was jeopardizing the safety of herself and others. She assaulted a faculty member and was escorted by the police to a juvenile detention center. After inpatient psychiatric treatment, I provided her school with her new diagnoses, DMDD and ASD, as well as a list of suggested accommodations provided to us. We were unaware of the process required for these new accommodations, which included a special behavior classroom to be incorporated, as it exceeded what was available under a 504 plan. Ultimately, her father and I, in addition to the school, concluded that she needed to be evaluated to provide the new accommodations that had been suggested for her disabilities. She now has an IEP and thrives in a specialized classroom with the sensory and behavioral accommodations helping her learn while staying safe.

Solution

Addressing the misunderstanding of a child's behavior requires education and awareness, especially in cases involving DMDD. Parents can play a vital role in this process by collaborating with school staff to ensure they have access to resources and training on DMDD and other mental health issues. Providing teachers with information about recognizing and responding to DMDD symptoms can prevent them from misinterpreting the child's actions as mere defiance. One of the most effective ways to support children with DMDD in the school environment is by developing an Individualized Education Plan (IEP) or a 504 plan. These plans can include specific accommodations tailored to the child's emotional and behavioral needs, such as allowing for breaks during the day, providing a quiet space to calm down, or offering alternative methods to communicate their emotions, like visual aids or written notes.

Additionally, regular professional development and training sessions for teachers and school staff on behavioral and mental health disorders can be highly beneficial. Such training can help them better understand the complexities of DMDD and equip them with strategies to support children effectively rather than resorting to punitive measures. Creating a supportive and informed school environment can foster positive relationships between educators and parents, ensuring the child receives the care and understanding they need.

Resolving Conflicts

When parents and school staff experience conflicts, both parties must focus on the child's best interests. Conflict can often emerge when misunderstandings occur, as in the case of Anika, whose behavioral outbursts were mistaken for defiance. In such situations, it's easy for emotions to escalate, leading to frustration on both sides. However, Anika's parents approached the issue with empathy and patience, choosing to explain their daughter's diagnosis of DMDD calmly. Instead of reacting defensively or aggressively, they took the time to educate Anika's teacher on DMDD, helping the teacher understand the root cause of Anika's behavior. This approach fostered an environment of understanding and cooperation, where the teacher became more aware of the disorder and was willing to collaborate on solutions.

By focusing on education and open communication, Anika's parents were able to resolve the conflict in a way that benefited their daughter. This example highlights how taking a constructive rather than confrontational approach can help de-escalate tensions and ensure that the child's needs remain at the forefront of discussions.

Solution

Adopting a collaborative, problem-solving approach is essential to constructively resolve conflicts between parents and schools. Both sides should actively listen to each other's perspectives and acknowledge the emotions that may arise during challenging conversations. Instead of focusing on blame or fault, the focus should be finding solutions that benefit the child's emotional and academic well-being. Parents can advocate effectively for their child by providing relevant documentation (a formal diagnosis, reports from mental health professionals, etc.) to help the school staff better understand their unique needs.

Additionally, parents can suggest strategies or accommodations that have been successful in other settings, such as at home or in therapy—these can create a practical foundation to build on. School staff should recognize that what works for most students may not necessarily work for a child with specific behavioral or emotional challenges and should remain open to adopting some approaches that have worked for the child's parents. By personalizing their approach and being accommodating to specific needs, school staff can create a more supportive learning environment that fosters the child's growth. Ultimately, maintaining open lines of communication and having a willingness to collaborate are critical to resolving conflicts and therefore to ensuring the child's emotional and academic success.

While parents of children with DMDD face unique challenges in building effective partnerships with schools, these barriers can be overcome through open communication, flexibility, and mutual understanding. By working together, parents and schools can create a supportive environment that allows children with DMDD to thrive academically and emotionally. Respectful, ongoing dialogue and a strong commitment to a child's best interests are the cornerstones of a successful partnership, and with patience and empathy, even difficult situations can be turned into opportunities for growth and collaboration.

Celebrating Successes Together

Celebrating a child's achievements, no matter how small, is an important part of building positive parent-school relationships. For children like Maya, Liam, and Anika, successes can range from attaining academic milestones to seeing improvements in emotional regulation. When parents and teachers celebrate these victories together, it reinforces the child's progress and motivates them to keep working on their emotional and academic growth.

Liam's teacher often sent home appreciative notes when he successfully used coping strategies during class. His parents then celebrated these moments with him, creating a positive feedback loop that encouraged further success. This kind of shared celebration helps strengthen the connections between home and school and reinforces the child's efforts.

Celebrating successes is related to spending part of the first parent-school meeting (as well as subsequent meetings) identifying and reinforcing a child's islands of competence. When a child is experiencing many challenges and their behaviors are problematic, it's easy for teachers and parents to spend the entire meeting talking about how best to "fix" the child's problems, with little discussion of the child's interests and strengths. Such a situation can create a negative climate that works against adults being more creative in considering strategies for helping that child develop a sense of competence and hope.

To address this tendency, one school principal developed a form that he asked his staff to complete prior to having any meeting about a student. At the top half of the page, teachers were asked to list the student's islands of competence, while the bottom half of the form requested teachers to list how they might use those strengths to help the student learn more effectively and feel more dignified in the school setting. The principal reported that including this one-page form in meetings led to more positive views of the student and more creative ways of helping the student to succeed and thrive in the school setting.

Building a Collaborative Community

For children with DMDD, having the support of a collaborative community is essential for their emotional well-being and development. Schools, families, and peers must work together to create a safe and nurturing environment where the child feels understood, accepted, and supported. Open communication between teachers, school counselors, and parents can help identify specific needs and tailor interventions that promote the child's academic and social success. Parent organizations such as PTAs can be critical in advocating for more robust mental health resources within schools. They can organize events that promote inclusivity and understanding, bringing an awareness of mental health challenges like DMDD and how they impact children. These efforts not only support the child but also educate the larger community, helping to reduce stigma and foster empathy among peers and educators.

For example, Anika's school held a mental health awareness week that included workshops for parents, teachers, and students. These sessions provided valuable information on emotional disorders like DMDD, helping to break down misunderstandings and encourage more open conversations about mental health. The activities that were organized for students (teambuilding exercises and discussions, to name a few) contributed to a more supportive atmosphere, allowing Anika's classmates to understand her condition better and demonstrate more compassion. Initiatives like this can play a pivotal role in creating an inclusive and supportive educational experience for children with DMDD and help them feel valued and heard.

The Lasting Impacts of a Strong Parent-School Partnership

The journeys of Emma, Maya, Liam, and Anika highlight the transformative power of collaboration between parents and schools. While the process may not always be free of challenges, the resulting partnership forms the foundation for children's academic achievement, emotional regulation, and personal growth. As advocates and partners, parents bring valuable insights into their child's behavior and needs, and at the same time, schools offer professional guidance and structured support. This teamwork helps create individualized strategies that foster academic progress and social and emotional well-being.

In the end, a solid parent-school partnership is more than beneficial—it's essential. Through consistent communication, mutual respect, and a shared commitment to children's wellbeing, parents and schools can work together to create an environment where every child can succeed regardless of their challenges. This partnership empowers children with DMDD to reach their full potential of personal and academic growth.

Chapter 13
Rising Through the Storm

In every storm, a force drives us to push through: hope. Hope is what serves as an anchor that keeps us from drifting into despair even when the winds howl and the seas rage. For children and families living with DMDD, the storm can be fierce and unrelenting—DMDD brings emotional volatility, frustration, and frequent outbursts, often creating an environment of unpredictability and tension. Yet amid these challenges, hope is the beacon of light that prevents families and children from losing their way. It unlocks the strength to navigate rough waters and offers stability when the journey feels overwhelming.

As the stories described in this book illustrate, it's always possible to rise through the storm. Each of these children and their families faced unique yet shared difficulties, from managing emotional turbulence to coping with the societal pressures surrounding mental health. But their stories also demonstrate that despite these adversities, with perseverance, guidance, and support, there *is* a path toward happiness and fulfillment.

This closing chapter explores the commonalities in these children's challenges, the strategies their families employed to overcome obstacles, and how hope and resilience—fueled by love and understanding—played a crucial role in paving the way for a brighter future for each child.

Similarities in Challenges: A Turbulent Journey

The journey for children with DMDD is marked by significant turmoil, both internally and externally. These children frequently experience extreme mood swings, explosive anger, and persistent irritability that can make even the most straightforward daily interactions feel like traversing a minefield. What might seem like a minor frustration to most can trigger overwhelming and unpredictable emotional outbursts in children with DMDD, making it difficult for them to maintain stability in social settings such as at home, at school, and in public spaces.

Their families find themselves on a parallel journey—they too must navigate an equally complex emotional landscape. Parents often feel isolated and overwhelmed as they search for effective ways to support their children; siblings may be frustrated or confused. Because they're frequently misunderstood by those around them, families may face judgment or unsolicited advice from others who don't understand the complexities of DMDD. Feelings of guilt can compound this isolation as parents question their abilities or wonder if they're doing enough to help their children. Uncertainty about the best course of action can weigh heavily on parents as they explore treatments, therapies, and strategies to manage their child's volatile emotions.

Across the stories of these children and parents, several recurring challenges stand out: stigma, difficulty in obtaining a correct diagnosis, the struggle to create treatment plans with effective interventions, and the toll that constant emotional upheaval takes on the entire family unit.

Early Signs of Emotional Dysregulation

Almost every child's story begins with early signs of distress. Ben, Jonas, Kellan, and Joseph exhibited intense irritability or behavioral challenges prior to preschool. This early emotional dysregulation—characterized by violent outbursts, rage, and an inability to selfsoothe—set the stage for years of turbulence. Their parents initially thought these behaviors were just part of the "terrible twos" and hoped they would pass with time. However, as each of these boys grew, their emotions escalated, leaving their parents physically and emotionally exhausted and unsure of how to cope.

Nathan's parents noticed his hypersensitivity and destructive behavior by the time he was three. His meltdowns over seemingly minor frustrations turned their household into a battleground, and the family began walking on eggshells, fearful of triggering his next emotional storm. At the same time, Patrick's early tantrums and aggression perplexed his adoptive parents, who had no frame of reference for understanding his intense emotional struggles. They searched for answers, but not only did traditional parenting techniques prove to ineffective, at times they exacerbated the situation.

These early signs often go unrecognized as being part of a broader disorder, leading to misdiagnoses and misguided treatments. Many parents are told that their children will "grow out of it" or that they need stricter discipline. Yet in these cases, beneath the surface something more complex is at play, something that requires a deeper understanding of the child's emotional worlds.

Struggles with Misdiagnoses and Inadequate Treatments

Misdiagnosis is a significant challenge for many families, often leading to prolonged struggles with incorrect treatments and worsening symptoms. For Nathan, the journey began with an autism spectrum disorder diagnosis, which was soon followed by a diagnosis of ADHD. However, rather than seeing improvements, his symptoms worsened, causing his family to question the accuracy of the diagnoses. The treatments Nathan was given seemed to aggravate his condition, leaving his parents confused and desperate for answers. Similarly, Ben experienced a complex diagnostic journey—he too was labeled with multiple conditions, including ADHD and PTSD. None of the various treatment plans Ben's family tried addressed the core issues driving his behaviors. It wasn't until his mother discovered the diagnosis of DMDD that they began to understand his underlying struggles.

Bella and Lizzie faced a similar path, with their diagnoses including anxiety, depression, and selective mutism. Each new diagnosis added another layer of complexity to their treatment plans, but nothing seemed to genuinely help—their family cycled through therapists and medications and only saw limited progress. Patrick, Joseph, and Kellan also received early ADHD diagnoses, but their violent outbursts remained unaddressed, leading to confusion and frustration for everyone involved. In all these cases, misdiagnoses contributed to years of ineffective treatments and amplified the emotional toll on families, who were left grappling with uncertainty and exhaustion.

Behavioral Outbursts and the Impacts on Family Life

For the families described in this book, violent outbursts and rages were a constant source of upheaval and fear for them and turned everyday life into a battleground. Kellan's episodes were incredibly destructive: he tore apart entire classrooms, he ran away from school, and he ultimately required hospitalization due to the severity of his behavior. And the chaos wasn't limited to school settings—in fact, Kellan's family bore the brunt of his unpredictable outbursts. His parents were constantly on edge, fearing what each day would bring. They described living with him as walking on eggshells, unsure when his next explosion would occur and how they would manage it without triggering a more severe reaction.

For Barry's mother, the fear was profoundly personal and invasive, as his explosions were so frequent and intense that she likened the situation to being trapped in an abusive relationship. His rages would leave her emotionally and physically drained; she never knew when the next confrontation would arise or how she could diffuse the situation. This constant state of anxiety eroded her sense of security as it made her home feel more like a war zone than a place of refuge.

For his part, Zack kicked his father in the head multiple times while being driven to the hospital. As they tried to manage Zack's behavior, his family also lived in fear.

Soon, they discovered that his younger sister Annie would also be diagnosed with DMDD.

In Bella and Lizzie's case, their outbursts were so severe that they physically altered the landscape of their home: they put holes in walls, shattered windows, broke doors, and smashed furniture. Their home reflected the inner turmoil these children were experiencing. Their parents were left with not only an overwhelming emotional toll but also the financial burden of frequent repairs; they often felt helpless in the face of such destructive behavior.

Similarly, Jonas exhibited frequent and unpredictable rages that escalated into both physical aggression and verbal abuse. His parents struggled to maintain control during his violent episodes, constantly fearing for the safety of everyone in the household.

The siblings of these children often felt overlooked and unsafe—they too were living in constant anxiety about what might happen next. Such explosive behaviors put immense pressure on family dynamics, as parents had to constantly balance the well-being of their child with DMDD against the emotional and physical needs of the rest of the family. The strain caused rifts between parents, increased sibling rivalry, and left families in a perpetual state of crisis management.

Isolation and Misunderstanding

Families of children with severe behavioral challenges like DMDD often experience both social and emotional isolation as they struggle to manage the complexities of their situation. The unpredictable nature of their children's behaviors can significantly strain social relationships. Friends and extended family members who may not fully understand or appreciate the depth of these challenges often distance themselves, either out of discomfort or misunderstanding. This can leave parents feeling as though they're navigating an overwhelming storm alone, without the support systems that many other families take for granted.

Public spaces that should offer respite or a chance for family bonding instead become battlegrounds filled with anxiety and dread. The unpredictability of the child's behavior can escalate quickly, turning what should be a simple, routine outing into a highly stressful situation. When meltdowns or disruptive behaviors occur in public, parents often feel judged by others, which only deepens their sense of isolation.

Jonas' mother shared how she often felt like a prisoner in her own home, unable to participate in everyday activities for fear of a behavioral outburst. Kellan's family faced repeated involvement with law enforcement due to his extreme behaviors, which compounded their stress and sense of helplessness. Zack and Annie's parents felt the loneliness that the diagnosis of DMDD caused and expressed how there was no escaping it, not even while they were on vacation. Such experiences create a profound sense of being misunderstood and further reinforce how isolated these families feel.

Rising Above the Challenges: Paths to Progress and Happiness

But still, despite the profound challenges these children and their families faced, many found a way to rise through the storm, demonstrating resilience and courage in the face of adversity. Their ability to overcome hardship can primarily be attributed to several shared factors that helped them persevere. Supportive community networks played a crucial role, providing emotional and practical assistance during tough times. Access to education and healthcare services also helped stabilize their lives and offered hope for a better future. And personal determination—coupled with love and encouragement from close family members—empowered them to push through obstacles and find success.

Finding the Right Diagnosis

For many families, the breakthrough in understanding their child's struggles comes when they finally receive a proper diagnosis of DMDD. After years of frustration, trial, and error with other diagnoses (ADHD, oppositional defiant disorder, even autism spectrum disorder), the identification of DMDD marks a turning point. This diagnosis opens the door to targeted treatments that most families have had to discover on their own; families also finally have access to interventions specifically designed to address the intense mood swings and emotional dysregulation that define DMDD. A diagnosis of DMDD allows parents and caregivers to better understand children's behavior and implement strategies that address the root cause of their distress rather than just the symptoms of it.

Ben's mother, for example, had been through a long and exhausting journey. She had tried various treatments, therapy options, and parenting strategies, all with little success. The diagnosis of DMDD finally made sense of her son's emotional volatility, and it led to an entirely new approach to his care. Similarly, Patrick's parents found themselves at their wits' end after having tried numerous interventions with no lasting results. It wasn't until they stumbled upon a Facebook support group that they heard about DMDD and the Matthews Protocol. This discovery was a game changer—it offered them hope and a path forward after years of confusion and dead ends. Ben's diagnosis brought not only clarity but also a sense of relief because they knew they weren't alone in their struggles.

Understanding DMDD provides families with a framework to guide their approach to treatments and day-to-day management. This new understanding is pivotal to improving their children's quality of life.

Effective Treatment and Medication

The key to transformation for many of the children we've profiled was the DMDD treatment protocol developed by Dr. Matthews. This protocol (which incorporates the use of anti-epileptic medications such as Trileptal® or Lamictal® and the antiviral drug amantadine, often used to treat Parkinson's symptoms) has proven to be life-changing for numerous families. By targeting the neurological and mood-related symptoms associated with DMDD, the Matthews Protocol offers children and their families a chance to regain control over their lives. The combination of anti-epileptic medication and amantadine has been shown to regulate emotional outbursts, stabilize moods, and reduce aggressive behaviors, making it possible for children to experience a higher quality of life.

> With each new medication we tried for our son, I was hopeful. I was hopeful with every new therapeutic approach, such as neurofeedback, biofeedback, diet, reduced screen time, tinctures, and herbs. With every new doctor, therapist, and even a two-week inpatient stay, I was hopeful. Hope started to dim when everything we tried had little or no success. I was not active on social media, so I was unaware of any support groups, and I felt alone on this journey. Then, one day, as I watched Dr. Larry Fisher's DMDD presentation on YouTube, my hope was reignited! It was as though this doctor was talking about my son and understood our plight. When Dr. Fisher explained how the aggressive children he and Dr. Dan Matthews worked with got better, I knew hope was alive. And that hope, combined with faith and love, led my son to healing.

The impact of the Matthews Protocol has transformed the lives of the children we've described and children worldwide. In the course of his practice, Dr. Matthews has seen many children and has also been treating children at a residential hospital with anti-epilepsy medication and amantadine since the 1970s. While he did not personally see the children profiled in this book, their parents were able to locate a doctor willing to use Dr. Matthews' protocol and be guided by his work and research.

> My son was seven when I first heard about Matthews Protocol and shared the information with his father. We were in the third year of seeking professional help for our son, who had been to more than half a dozen doctors and therapists and had spent time in a psychiatric unit. My son's father responded, 'So what makes this time different? Why is this time the answer when nothing we've done in the past has worked?' I told him, 'Just because nothing in the past has helped doesn't mean this won't.' Now, my son has been stable for over six years, no longer needs his IEP for behavioral support, yet hasn't forgotten how difficult his life used to be. He wants other children with DMDD never to give up hope. Things can get better!

Nathan and Joseph, for instance, experienced a dramatic reduction in their frequent, uncontrollable rages once they were placed on the protocol. Their parents—who had long struggled to find a solution for their sons' volatile behavior—finally began to experience a sense of hope for his future. The transformation was equally profound for Ben, Joseph, Barry, and Zack, all of whom had previously been violent and brutal to manage. After a few months of treatment, these children became respectful and thriving teenagers, much to the relief of their families. Similarly, Kellan, Patrick, Annie, Ethan, and Emma significantly improved their behavior when placed on the Matthews Protocol. These children experienced a newfound ability to manage their emotions, allowing them to interact more positively with their families and peers. For all of these families, the DMDD medication protocol provided the long-hoped breakthrough they needed to move forward with their lives.

Supportive Relationships

A recurring theme in these stories is the vital role played by a supportive adult figure— often a parent, coach, or therapist—who refused to give up on the child. Ben's basketball coach is an excellent example of someone who not only recognized his potential but also provided him with a lifeline that helped transform the course of his life. Annie's mother became a pillar of strength, constantly reminding her daughter of her inherent courage and refusing to allow her struggles to define her. She didn't just offer emotional support, she also gave her daughter practical help that made a world of difference. In our strength-based model, we refer to these people as "charismatic adults," defined by the late psychologist Julius Segal as adults from whom "children gather strength."

> Authors like Mona Delahooke's *Brain-Body Parenting,* and Robyn Gobbel's *Raising Kids with Big Baffling Behaviors* discuss behavior from a body-brain approach, that focuses on the nervous system to change behavior. I've found these books to be good resources with tips to help calm my daughter's big emotions that DMDD brings to the table. I've started to notice when she's irritable, if certain foods help her more than others, like crunchy nacho chips, cold ice-cream or something sweet. Thinking of emotions in terms of the nervous system has made me implement a few of my own ideas, like offering reflexology, a valuable tool for calming my daughter before sleep. Reflexology engages the nervous system and promotes relaxation, and while this helps my child relax enough to fall asleep, it is also a special bonding time between mother and daughter. That time together reassures her that even though she may have had a difficult day handling her emotions, she is truly loved.

For many children with DMDD, their parents are instrumental in their recovery journeys. Despite facing overwhelming challenges, charismatic adults like the parents we've talked about in this book exhibit unwavering love and determination. Ben's mother, for instance, took the bold step of removing him from a psychiatric hospital where he would have become a ward of the state, and she did so against medical advice—she trusted her own instincts about his wellbeing. Meanwhile, Jonas' mother tirelessly fought to ensure that he received the proper treatment; she became his strongest advocate in the face of adversity.

Personal Growth and Transformation

As these children received the proper treatment and support, many experienced remarkable personal growth that exceeded all initial expectations. Jonas, once consumed by uncontrollable rage and frustration, became a dedicated and enthusiastic member of his school's robotics team. What had once seemed impossible—his ability to work collaboratively and calmly with others—became a reality as he formed meaningful friendships and embraced his new role. His participation in group activities fostered better social connections and built up his confidence, giving him a sense of purpose and belonging. Barry, who had once seemed destined for a life filled with escalating crises and constant turmoil, began to show remarkable signs of development and functionality. The chaos that had previously defined his life started to subside, replaced by moments of stability and growth. With every step forward, his family's hope for his future deepened as they began to see a path filled with the kinds of possibilities they had once thought were out of reach.

Through the right combination of therapies, support, and perseverance, Jonas and Barry found their way to a place where they could thrive, bringing newfound optimism to their families and communities. Bella and Lizzie—whose destructive behaviors had once torn their family apart—now exhibit emotional stability thanks to the Matthews Protocol. Where Patrick had struggled to make friends and control his impulses, he's now a leader in his youth group and participates in a travel lacrosse team. Despite having been previously trapped in a cycle of rage and despair, these children found their way to a brighter future through persistence, treatment, and support.

Learning When to Act

As much as the parents we've profiled have valued the hierarchy of strategies they've learned, there have been moments when actions had to precede words. Over time, they've meticulously built a toolbox of techniques that range from gentle persuasion to collaborative problem-solving. They have practiced restraint, believing that calm, reflective responses would yield the best results. However, in moments of crisis—when tensions were high or when their child's immediate well-being was at stake—swift, decisive action was essential. They realized that no amount of dialogue could replace the necessity of acting quickly to protect or redirect their child during dangerous or highly emotional situations.

In these moments, parents understood that although their well-rehearsed words were valuable in calmer situations, sometimes those words needed to take a back seat to instinct and decisive intervention. For instance, when a child was engaging in harmful behavior or an emotional meltdown had escalated into something more volatile, there was no time to analyze the situation in depth or deliberate over which strategy would be most effective. Instead, immediate and firm action was required to stop the behavior and ensure everyone's safety.

But these instances didn't contradict the careful strategies the parents had developed— they reinforced the parents' understanding of the balance between thoughtful responses and timely interventions. They learned that sometimes words could wait. In these situations, the priority became acting quickly to diffuse a situation and *then* returning to process and reflect once the crisis had passed.

By recognizing when action was needed over conversation, these parents gained confidence in their ability to protect their child and restore calm. Importantly, they also held space for communication once the immediate danger or heightened emotions had subsided, demonstrating their commitment to maintaining a healthy relationship with their child.

Resilient Children with DMDD

At the heart of every success story lies the unwavering belief that change is possible even when circumstances seem overwhelmingly complex. No matter how fierce the storm is, there's always the hope that the clouds will eventually part and the sun will shine again! This mindset of hope is not only inspiring but essential for children with DMDD and their families. Living with DMDD often means confronting intense emotional turmoil and behavioral challenges that can leave both the child and their loved ones feeling helpless or defeated—the belief that things can improve is the very foundation of resilience.

The journey toward emotional regulation and well-being requires not only treatment but also the hope that progress is achievable. Families must value and hold on to this belief, even during the most trying times, as it sustains them through setbacks and frustrations. Hope allows them to seek new therapies, advocate for their children, and make progress despite the obstacles they may face. This hope-driven inner strength leads to breakthroughs and personal growth. With the right mindset and support, families and children can learn how to navigate even the darkest of storms and can emerge from them all the stronger, filled with the faith that yes, there *will* be brighter days ahead.

Embracing a Growth Mindset

For children with DMDD, the journey to emotional stability is often complex and unpredictable. Unlike a smooth, linear path, progress frequently ebbs and flows, with periods of calm usually interrupted by emotional outbursts or regressions. These setbacks can be incredibly frustrating for both the child and their caregivers, leading to moments of doubt and uncertainty about whether real progress is being made. Parents may question if all the hard work is worth it, particularly when a child who seems to be improving suddenly reverts to old behaviors. However, it's essential to understand that these fluctuations are a natural part of the emotional development process for children with DMDD. Especially in the context of a disorder characterized by severe mood dysregulation, a child's emotional growth rarely follows a perfect or predictable trajectory. Setting unrealistic expectations for consistent, flawless improvement can lead to disappointment, discouragement, and a sense of failure for the child *and* their support network.

All of this is why adopting a growth mindset can be profoundly empowering for both the child and their caregivers. A growth mindset encourages the belief that setbacks are not signs of failure but rather opportunities for learning and development. When an emotional episode occurs, instead of viewing it as a regression, families can reframe the situation as a moment to build resilience, strengthen coping mechanisms, and gain deeper insights into the child's emotional triggers. Caregivers play a crucial role in this process and provide much-needed support and guidance. For instance, a particularly difficult outburst may highlight environmental or psychological triggers that had previously gone unnoticed, offering new perspectives on how to better manage and anticipate emotional responses in the future. This shift in perception allows for more constructive responses to challenges and fosters a sense of hope and perseverance even in difficult times.

Furthermore, a growth mindset promotes patience and persistence, two qualities that are essential for both caregivers and children. It reminds them that progress is often slow and incremental but that every small victory represents meaningful progress. Even the tiniest steps forward (like managing one emotional episode better than the last) can be celebrated as signs of growth. Over time, these small steps accumulate into significant milestones, leading children with DMDD toward greater emotional stability. This mindset not only helps children cope with the daily challenges of DMDD, it also equips them with essential life skills such as selfawareness, emotional regulation, and resilience.

Focusing on What **Can** *Be Controlled*

One of the critical characteristics of a resilient mindset is the ability to focus on what *can* be controlled, especially in challenging or unpredictable situations. For children diagnosed with DMDD, this concept becomes particularly important.

These children often experience intense emotions and difficulty with managing their behaviors, and external factors beyond their control can exacerbate their challenges. However, by learning to focus on what they *can* control—such as their emotional responses and how they manage their behavior—children can develop the skills they need to navigate their environment more effectively. This approach helps them regulate their emotions and empowers them to take ownership of their actions, creating a foundation for long-term success in both personal and academic settings.

Patrick's story is a powerful illustration of the significance of resilience. He initially struggled with emotional outbursts and behavioral issues that impacted his ability to function in school and social settings, but with the support of an Individualized Education Program and the proper medication, he was able to develop tools and strategies that allowed him to manage his emotions more effectively at school. By applying these tools, Patrick gradually gained control over his behaviors, which enabled him to thrive. His academic performance improved and his ability to engage positively with his peers grew stronger, demonstrating the profound impact of focusing on what *can* be controlled.

A note: it's also very important for parents and other caregivers to develop personal control. While parents don't have any control over their child having a diagnosis of DMDD, they *do* have more control (more than they may realize!) over their attitude and their responses to their child's struggles. With a more controlled, positive attitude, parents can more effectively assess their child's situation and apply interventions that will help their child become more resilient.

The Role of Supportive Adults

Children with DMDD cannot meet the challenges of managing their emotions and behaviors on their own. That's why the presence of a supportive adult—whether a parent, teacher, coach, or therapist—is essential for their success and emotional development. These adults play a pivotal role in providing the hope, encouragement, and guidance that children need to persevere through the difficulties that often accompany DMDD. Their belief in the child's potential and their consistent emotional support serves as a foundation for growth and resilience. Supportive adults aren't just passive figures, they help children find strategies to cope with their emotional challenges and advocate for key resources to promote their well-being.

These "charismatic adults" provide practical support and are an inspirational presence in a child's life. A charismatic adult believes deeply in the child's potential and often sees possibilities where others might only see obstacles. Their unwavering dedication, positive energy, and strong advocacy can transform the child's emotional well-being and development. In the lives of Annie, Ben, and Jonas, for example, such figures proved to be pivotal. Whether it was Ben's coach, Annie's mother, or Jonas' parents, these charismatic adults helped them weather the storms of DMDD and emerge stronger.

The Power of Hope

Hope is the driving force behind resilience, particularly for families grappling with the challenges of DMDD. In the face of intense emotional storms, frequent outbursts, and unpredictable behaviors, hope becomes the anchor that keeps families grounded. It sustains them during the darkest and most trying times, encouraging them to search for answers even when the future seems bleak. Hope propels them forward, offering a sense of possibility that change and improvement are achievable. For families facing DMDD, hope is often what leads them to advocate for their children, seek out new treatments, and fight for the resources that can make a meaningful difference in their lives.

This belief in a better future is exemplified in the stories of Ben's mother, Nathan's parents, and Kellan's family. Despite hearing from professionals that their children might never improve or be able to manage their emotions, these families never wavered. Their hope persisted even in the face of discouraging predictions. It was their unwavering hope—combined with an eventual correct diagnosis and appropriate treatment plans—that paved the way for their children's transformation.

For Ben, Nathan, and Kellan, the hope their families had led to remarkable progress. Once they were armed with the right strategies—whether those were through therapy, medication, or behavioral interventions—these children began to develop tools to manage their emotions and behaviors. Their progress wasn't immediate nor was it without challenges, but the hope their families maintained provided the strength the children needed to keep pushing forward. Hope allowed them to believe that yes, improvement *was* possible even when they were faced with setbacks. In the end, hope paired with proper support and treatment allowed these children to find new levels of success and well-being. Without hope, their journeys might have looked very different.

The Dreams and Wishes of Parents

Parents of children diagnosed with DMDD want the same things that *all* parents want for their children: happiness, success, and strong social connections. While their dreams are shaped by the unique emotional and behavioral challenges that come with DMDD, their hopes remain the same. These parents also long for stability, emotional balance, and resilience as their children face life's emotional ups and downs. Of course, their journey may involve navigating intense emotional outbursts, irritability, and frustration, making resilience and emotional growth even more essential for their children's well-being.

As they continue to assess their children, many parents begin to see their role as managing their children's DMDD symptoms rather than nurturing their general well-being. Helping children regulate their emotions can be exhausting and can often leave parents questioning their ability to foster the long-term resilience they know is necessary for their children's future success. This added layer of complexity shifts parental expectations toward a more specific and targeted approach that focuses on building emotional regulation skills alongside pursuing traditional parenting goals like academic success and social development.

Parents may struggle with how they can and should promote resilience in their children when emotional regulation seems so elusive. The typical advice to encourage their children to engage in problem-solving or to persevere despite obstacles can feel inadequate when children are faced with frequent and intense emotional outbursts. When a child with DMDD gets so frustrated over seemingly minor challenges, parents may find that traditional approaches like reasoning or offering solutions are ineffective, a result that often leaves them feeling helpless. For their children with DMDD, parents realize, resilience isn't just about coping with adversity but also learning to manage their emotional responses in the first place.

For this reason, many parents of children with DMDD turn to therapeutic techniques designed to address emotional dysregulation, such as cognitive-behavioral strategies or mindfulness practices. These methods are seen as tools to help manage immediate behavioral challenges; they're foundational for children to develop the resilience they'll need to face future stressors. While all parents hope that their children will be successful, parents of children with DMDD may focus more heavily on building emotional endurance and providing their children with coping mechanisms that allow them to thrive despite their mood disorder. In this context, resilience is the cornerstone of parenting—it guides every decision, practice, and interaction.

Words for the Professionals Who Work with Children with DMDD and Their Families

To the mental health, medical, and educational professionals reading this, your role in supporting children with DMDD cannot be overstated. You are in a position to serve as a charismatic adult for children with DMDD and their families. As you now know, DMDD is a condition characterized by severe and recurrent temper outbursts, irritability, and mood instability that can disrupt a child's ability to function academically, socially, and emotionally. It is *not* a problem of bad behavior, poor parenting, or spoiled children. The children and families dealing with DMDD face a unique set of challenges, and your expertise, compassion, and collaboration are crucial in guiding them toward a path of hope and healing.

For mental health professionals, your role in early identification, accurate diagnosis, and ongoing treatment is essential. Children with DMDD often experience significant emotional distress, and without proper intervention, they are at risk of long-term difficulties, including issues with peer relationships, academic achievement, and self-esteem. You are tasked with providing therapeutic tools and strategies to help these children to manage intense emotions and with offering a space for children and their families to feel understood and supported.

Medical professionals play an equally important role, because for many children, a combination of medication and behavioral therapy proves to be the most effective. Your careful evaluation and treatment planning can significantly reduce the frequency and intensity of emotional outbursts, enabling children to regulate their emotions and behaviors more effectively. Your guidance in educating families about treatment options, potential side effects, and the importance of consistency in care can help alleviate fear and uncertainty.

Meanwhile, educators are on the front line, able to observe the impact of DMDD in the classroom (perhaps on a daily basis). Your ability to implement accommodations, provide structure, and work closely with parents and specialists can make a profound difference in a child's ability to succeed academically and socially. Your patience, understanding, and willingness to collaborate are vital in creating an environment where children with DMDD can thrive.

Together, your efforts create a robust network of support that allows children with DMDD to lead fulfilling and productive lives. Combining your expertise and compassionate care, you help these children develop tools to manage their emotions, navigate social relationships, and succeed academically. Your nonjudgmental approach with parents allows them to feel that they are not "bad" parents and that they did not "cause" their child's DMDD. This compassionate mindset is an essential component of your interactions with parents. Through your collaboration and dedication, you offer them a brighter future, one where their children can reach their full potential despite the challenges they face. Your role is instrumental in empowering children and their families; you instill hope that improvement is possible and that their journey will be one of resilience and progress.

Rising Through the Storm

The stories described in this book aren't just tales of survival—they're stories of triumph. Although these children and their families faced incredible challenges, they found a path to happiness and success through knowledge, resilience, hope, and the proper support. Their journeys illustrate the power of a resilient mindset and the importance of believing in a brighter future no matter how fierce the storm may become. While the storm may be extended and turbulent, with the right mindset and support, it *is* possible to rise through it. The future is not fixed! On the contrary, it's full of possibilities. With hope as their guide, these children and their families are finding their way to calmer seas and sunny skies.

The stories we've shared with you are proof that the future is not written in stone despite the unpredictability and hardships brought on by DMDD. Every setback and every challenge these children faced was met with determination, a willingness to fight, and the unwavering support of loved ones and professionals. In addressing their obstacles head-on, these families have demonstrated that DMDD does not define a child's potential. Their successes remind us that progress may be within reach given knowledge, proper care, therapeutic interventions, and emotional support.

In the end, the triumph these children have achieved is a beacon of hope for all children and families struggling with DMDD. Their victories serve as a potent reminder that no matter how overwhelming challenges may seem, progress and growth *can* happen. Through proper support, therapy, and unwavering dedication, children with DMDD can develop the tools they need to manage their emotions and navigate life successfully. Even the darkest storms will pass—these children and their loved ones can build a brighter, more promising future through persistence, love, and understanding.

Their journeys inspire others to hold on, seek help, and believe in the possibility of transformation. The families you've read about are lighting the way for more families to follow.

Appendix A

Effective Strategies for Conflict Resolution in Children

Helping children navigate emotional and behavioral challenges, such as refusal (e.g., not doing chores, resisting bedtime, or avoiding homework), disappointment, frustration (often linked to stress and heightened sensory sensitivity), or even outbursts, requires thoughtful strategies that foster understanding, empathy, and resilience. Traditional reactions—like yelling, dismissing their feelings, or imposing immediate punishments—often escalate conflicts, hindering a child's ability to self-regulate and learn problem-solving skills. Instead, adopting supportive and constructive approaches helps encourage emotional growth and better conflict resolution.

For example, when a child refuses to perform a task, the instinct to demand compliance or threaten punishment can backfire, reinforcing resistance. Alternatively, explaining the importance of the task and providing structured choices (e.g., "You can start now or in 10 minutes") can empower the child to cooperate without feeling cornered, and, similarly, validating feelings when disappointed or frustrated helps them feel heard. It builds trust, while strategies like offering sensory tools or calm spaces can help them regulate emotions effectively.

Outbursts, often stemming from an overwhelmed emotional state, require a different approach. During these moments, the brain's prefrontal cortex—responsible for reasoning—shuts down, making reasoning ineffective. Giving the child space while maintaining visual contact allows their brain to return to baseline before engaging in problem-solving or comfort. In extreme cases where safety is a concern, external intervention may be necessary.

This table provides practical strategies tailored to three primary environments—home, school, and the playground—to address such behaviors constructively. Each scenario outlines common ineffective responses, suggests alternative actions, and provides backup strategies for flexibility. These methods foster a calm, empathetic environment where children feel respected and capable, empowering them to build self-regulation skills and engage in healthier, more constructive interactions.

Home strategies		
What doesn't work	Instead, try	If it fails, try
Yelling or raising your voice	Use a calm, neutral tone and clearly state expectations.	Take a break yourself, then re-engage once both parties are calm.
Ignoring a child's feelings	Acknowledge and validate their emotions.	Suggest a quiet activity or sensory tool to help them self-soothe.
Giving immediate consequences without explanation	Explain the reason for the consequence and offer a chance to try again.	Use logical consequences that focus on learning rather than punishment.
Dismissing a child's request without hearing them out	Listen fully and offer choices when possible.	Rephrase their request to ensure understanding, then gently repeat the available options.
Punishing for not finishing a task	Offer support, break tasks into smaller steps, or set a timer for focused effort.	Introduce a reward system that celebrates small achievements to build motivation.
Responding to whining with "stop whining"	Acknowledge their need and encourage a more effective way to communicate.	Set clear guidelines for asking for help, practicing these skills together when both parties are calm.
Solving every problem for the child	Encourage problem-solving by asking guiding questions.	Model a similar situation and invite them to brainstorm solutions together.
Reacting negatively to emotional outbursts	Practice calm breathing with them and give them space.	Provide a quiet corner or calming activity like drawing to help them regulate their emotions.
Criticizing their lack of effort	Praise their attempts and encourage incremental progress.	Set smaller, achievable steps and celebrate each success.
Making decisions for capable children	Allow choices within set limits to encourage independence.	Offer limited, structured options to help them feel in control while guiding their decisions.

School strategies		
What doesn't work	Instead, try	If it fails, try
Raising your voice in response to defiance	Speak calmly, using a non-threatening tone.	Allow silence for a moment before re-engaging with a soft prompt or question.
Ignoring students struggling with directions	Offer a private reminder or additional support.	Provide visual aids or written instructions for clarity.
Punishing disruptive behavior without understanding the cause	Discuss the root of the behavior privately with the student.	Involve a counselor or support staff to explore underlying issues.
Enforcing rules without explanation	Explain the purpose of rules calmly and neutrally.	Reinforce with relatable examples of how rules benefit everyone.

(continued)

Appendix A

School strategies

What doesn't work	Instead, try	If it fails, try
Reacting to negativity with frustration	Model positive communication, even in challenging situations.	Take a deep breath and ask how you can support or help the student.
Blaming students for incomplete work	Ask if there's a specific difficulty and offer solutions.	Use a check-in system or involve parents to help monitor progress.
Assuming all students understand expectations	Clearly outline expectations and provide frequent reminders.	Post visual cues or reminders around the classroom for reinforcement.
Insisting on immediate apologies	Allow time for the student to calm down before discussing apologies.	Use restorative conversations later to reflect and learn from the incident.
Giving instructions only once	Repeat calmly, using simple language for clarity.	Implement a buddy system, pairing students to help each other with compliance.
Reacting defensively to fairness complaints	Listen and validate concerns before explaining decisions.	Create a suggestion box for students to share concerns respectfully.

Playground strategies

What doesn't work	Instead, try	If it fails, try
Breaking up conflicts without listening to both sides	Allow each child to explain their perspective.	Facilitate peer mediation with adult guidance.
Ignoring signs of frustration during play	Intervene gently to ask how the child feels and offer support.	Suggest a break or another activity until calmness is restored.
Forcing children to "just get along"	Guide a discussion to resolve disagreements respectfully.	Use a simple conflict resolution script, allowing each child to speak in turn.
Dismissing complaints about teasing	Encourage assertive responses and offer specific phrases they can use.	Follow up to ensure they feel safe and supported.
Expecting all children to play the same way	Provide options for diverse play styles and ensure inclusivity.	Offer quiet spaces or different play materials to accommodate various interests.
Allowing rough play without boundaries	Clearly set boundaries and ensure everyone knows the rules.	Pause the game to discuss rules collectively and restart only when calm.
Focusing solely on winning in games	Promote cooperative games, emphasizing teamwork over competition.	Rotate roles or responsibilities to balance competitiveness.
Enforcing play without breaks	Incorporate time-outs for cooling down as part of playtime.	Rotate activities to ensure a mix of high- and low-pressure play options.

By prioritizing empathy, patience, and flexibility, caregivers and educators can create environments where children feel safe expressing their emotions, learning from their experiences, and becoming resilient individuals. Empathy helps adults view situations from the child's perspective, acknowledging their struggles without judgment. This fosters trust and opens communication channels, enabling children to feel heard and understood even during moments of conflict. For example, rather than dismissing a child's frustration over a seemingly minor issue, a caregiver can validate their feelings, showing that their emotions matter and providing reassurance that challenges can be addressed together.

Patience is equally critical, as behavioral growth often happens gradually. Children need time to process their emotions and practice new skills. When caregivers remain calm and composed, even during setbacks, they model emotional regulation, teaching children to manage their reactions constructively. Flexibility complements these efforts by allowing adults to adapt their approaches to each child's unique needs and the context of the situation. A one-size-fits-all solution rarely works in complex emotional or behavioral scenarios.

These strategies help children manage immediate conflicts and lay the groundwork for long-term development. Children learn to navigate challenges, build self-confidence, and form positive relationships with consistent support, fostering harmony across home, school, and play settings.

Appendix B

Understanding Your Child's Rights Under IDEIA and Section 504/ADA: A Guide for Parents

Sam Goldstein, Ph.D.

Navigating the educational rights and protections for children with disabilities can be overwhelming for parents. The Individuals with Disabilities Education Improvement Act (IDEIA), Section 504 of the Rehabilitation Act, and the Americans with Disabilities Act (ADA) are federal laws designed to protect these children. This brief guide provides a detailed understanding of each law, its similarities and differences, and the assessment and eligibility determination processes. It is not meant to offer legal advice.

Table of Contents

IDEIA vs. Section 504/ADA: An Overview
Similarities Between IDEIA and Section 504/ADA
Critical Differences Between IDEIA and Section 504/ADA
Assessment and Eligibility Determination
The Individualized Education Program (IEP) Process
Section 504 Accommodation Plans
What Parents Can Do: Advocacy Tips and Resources
References

IDEIA vs. Section 504/ADA: An Overview

IDEIA (Individuals with Disabilities Education Improvement Act) is a federal law providing specific protections to students with disabilities. First enacted in 1975 and reauthorized in 2004, IDEIA requires public schools to offer a "Free Appropriate Public Education" (FAPE) in the "Least Restrictive Environment" (LRE) for children with disabilities who qualify for special education services. It covers children ages 3 to 21 who meet certain eligibility criteria based on specific categories of disabilities, such as autism, learning disabilities, and speech/language impairments.

Section 504 of the Rehabilitation Act of 1973 and the Americans with Disabilities Act (ADA), in contrast, are civil rights laws that protect individuals with disabilities from discrimination—section 504 applies to any program or activity receiving federal financial assistance, including public schools. At the same time, ADA extends to all public and private schools (with some exceptions). Section 504/ADA protects students who may not qualify under IDEIA but still have a physical or mental impairment that substantially limits one or more major life activities, such as learning, speaking, or walking.

Similarities Between IDEIA and Section 504/ADA

Both IDEIA and Section 504/ADA aim to ensure that children with disabilities receive equitable access to education. However, they achieve this through different mechanisms:

- Protection Against Discrimination: Both laws prohibit discrimination against students with disabilities and mandate reasonable accommodations to ensure equal access to educational programs.
- Parental Involvement: Parents have the right to be involved in their child's educational planning, regardless of whether the child is served under IDEIA or Section 504. This includes meeting participation, access to records, and the right to request evaluations.
- Access to FAPE: Although IDEIA explicitly defines and mandates FAPE, Section 504 also requires schools to provide free and appropriate public education, though with less specificity regarding service delivery and individualized instruction.
- Procedural Safeguards: Both laws include procedural safeguards to protect students' and parents' rights. These can involve dispute resolution processes, such as due process hearings and the right to file complaints if parents feel their child's rights are violated.

Appendix B 231

Critical Differences Between IDEIA and Section 504/ADA

Eligibility Criteria
- IDEIA: Only students with disabilities falling under one of 13 specific categories (e.g., autism, emotional disturbance, learning disabilities) are eligible. The disability must also adversely impact the child's educational performance, necessitating specialized instruction.
- Section 504/ADA: Eligibility is broader, covering any student with a physical or mental impairment that substantially limits a significant life activity, such as learning. This law does not require an adverse impact on educational performance or a need for specialized instruction, making it more accessible to students with a range of disabilities.

Services Provided
- IDEIA: Requires an Individualized Education Program (IEP), a legally binding document detailing the student's unique needs, goals, and the specific special education services the school will provide.
- Section 504/ADA: Uses a 504 Plan, which typically includes accommodations rather than specialized instruction. These accommodations could consist of physical accessibility modifications, extended time on tests, or seating arrangements. A 504 Plan is generally less comprehensive and legally binding than an IEP.

Funding and Accountability
- IDEIA: Schools receive federal funding to provide the services outlined in students' IEPs. As a result, there are strict compliance requirements, and the federal government regularly monitors states.
- Section 504/ADA: These laws do not provide additional federal funding to schools for accommodations or services. Schools must accommodate students without federal assistance, although failure to comply can result in federal complaints and investigations.

Protections and Rights
- IDEIA: This encompasses a more extensive set of procedural safeguards and due process rights, such as formal evaluations every three years, progress reports, and reevaluations if needs change.
- Section 504/ADA: Has fewer procedural requirements. For example, evaluations are less frequent and less comprehensive. Changes to a 504 Plan can often be made without a formal meeting or extensive documentation.

Assessment and Eligibility Determination

IDEIA Assessment and Eligibility

Under IDEIA, schools are required to conduct a complete and individualized evaluation before determining eligibility for special education services. The assessment process involves:

- Referral: Parents, teachers, or other professionals can request an assessment if they suspect a child has a disability.
- Evaluation: A multidisciplinary team conducts a comprehensive review, considering factors such as academic performance, cognitive abilities, and social-emotional skills.
- Eligibility Determination: The team, including the parents, reviews evaluation data to determine if the child meets one of the 13 disability categories. If eligible, an IEP meeting is held within 30 days to develop a plan tailored to the child's needs.

Section 504/ADA Assessment and Eligibility

Section 504 eligibility criteria are broader and less formal:

- Referral: Parents or school staff can make a referral if they believe the child has an impairment affecting major life activities.
- Evaluation: The evaluation process needs to be more comprehensive than IDEIA's and may include observations, academic records, and input from teachers or medical professionals.
- Eligibility Determination: If the evaluation shows that the child has a disability substantially limiting a significant life activity, the school creates a 504 Plan outlining the specific accommodations needed.

The Individualized Education Program (IEP) Process

For students who qualify under IDEIA, the IEP is a critical document that guides their education. The IEP process involves several steps:

- Developing the IEP: An IEP team, which includes the child's parents, special and general education teachers, a school administrator, and specialists, collaborates to develop a comprehensive plan.
- Defining Goals: The IEP includes measurable annual goals detailing specific skills and competencies the child should achieve.
- Services and Accommodations: The IEP specifies the special education services, related services (e.g., speech therapy), and accommodations the student will receive.

Appendix B

- Progress Monitoring: Schools must regularly monitor progress toward IEP goals and report it to parents.
- Annual Review: The IEP is reviewed at least annually to make necessary adjustments based on the child's progress and changing needs.

Section 504/ADA Accommodation Plans

For students who qualify under Section 504, a 504 Plan provides accommodations to support equal access to education:

- Developing the 504 Plan: Typically, a school team collaborates with parents to create a plan that meets the child's needs. Although formalized meetings are not always required, parental input is crucial.
- Accommodations: The 504 Plan includes accommodations based on the child's specific needs, such as preferential seating, extended test time, or modified assignments.
- Flexibility: Unlike an IEP, the 504 Plan does not usually require an annual review. However, schools often review these plans periodically to ensure continued appropriateness.

What Parent Can Do: Advocacy Tips and Resources

Navigating IDEIA and Section 504/ADA protections requires active parental advocacy:

- Request Evaluations in Writing: Whether pursuing an IEP under IDEIA or a 504 Plan, a written request for evaluation can help expedite the process.
- Understand Your Rights: Familiarize yourself with procedural safeguards, such as the right to appeal decisions, file complaints, and attend all relevant meetings.
- Documentation is Key: Keep records of meetings, correspondence, and evaluations to ensure accountability and to assist if disputes arise.
- Stay Informed: Educational rights for children with disabilities are continually evolving. Organizations like the PACER Center (pacer.org) and the U.S. Department of Education (ed.gov) provide resources and updates.
- Seek Support: Many states have local advocacy organizations that offer guidance, and some provide legal resources to support parents through the evaluation and plan development process.

References

U.S. Department of Education, Office of Special Education Programs. "IDEIA – Individuals with Disabilities Education Act." https://sites.ed.gov/idea/.

U.S. Department of Education, Office for Civil Rights. "Section 504 of the Rehabilitation Act of 1973." https://www2.ed.gov/about/offices/list/ocr/504faq.html.

Resources

Several organizations provide invaluable support, services, and information when seeking mental health resources. Each group offers a unique approach to addressing mental health challenges, from advocacy and education to direct intervention.

Advocacy and General Mental Health Support

Depression and Bipolar Support Alliance (DBSA) focuses on empowering individuals living with mood disorders by offering peer-based wellness resources, tools, and support groups. (https://www.dbsalliance.org/)

The National Institute of Mental Health (NIMH) is a leading governmental body that conducts mental health research and disseminates evidence-based information to the public. (https://www.nimh.nih.gov/)

Anxiety and Depression Association of America (ADAA) is committed to preventing, treating, and curing anxiety and depression through education, practice, and research. (https://www.adaa.org/)

Focused Mental Health Initiatives

DMDD.org specializes in providing resources and support for families and individuals managing Disruptive Mood Dysregulation Disorder (DMDD). (https://www.dmdd.org/)

National Alliance on Mental Illness (NAMI) offers advocacy, education, and support for individuals and families affected by mental illness, aiming to build better lives for those in need. (https://www.nami.org/)

Camber Mental Health focuses on behavioral health services for children and adolescents, promoting early intervention and specialized care. (https://www.cambermentalhealth.org/)

Youth and Family Mental Health

Child Mind Institute is dedicated to transforming the lives of children and families struggling with mental health disorders and learning difficulties through research and clinical care. (https://childmind.org/resources/)

The National Association for Children's Behavioral Health (NACBH) provides resources. (https://www.nacbh.org)

The Kid Mental Health Foundation empowers children and their families with educational tools to promote mentail wellness. (https://www.kidsmentalhealthfoundation.org/)

Specialized Organizations

International Bipolar Foundation (IBPF) offers education, support, and awareness programs to help those impacted by bipolar disorder. (https://ibpf.org/)

International OCD Foundation (IOCDF) provides resources to individuals and families affected by obsessive-compulsive disorder and related disorders. (https://iocdf.org/)

Autism Speaks supports individuals with autism through advocacy, education, and resources aimed at improving quality of life. (https://www.autismspeaks.org)

Revolutionize DMDD (http//:www.RDMDD.org) is a transformative initiative dedicated to advance understanding, support, and innovative treatments for children and families of Disruptive Mood Dysregulation Disorder (DMDD).

MindUp, The Goldie Hawn Foundation (http://www.mindup.org), provides evidence-based programs that equip children, educators, and families with mindfulness and social-emotional tools to enhance focus, resilience, and overall well-being.

LGBTQ+ and Social Justice Mental Health Advocacy

The Trevor Project is the leading organization providing crisis intervention and suicide prevention services to LGBTQ+ youth. (https://www.thetrevorproject.org/)

BEAM (Black Emotional and Mental Health Collective) focuses on mental health and healing justice for Black communities through education, advocacy, and culture change. (https://www.beam.community/)

Substance Use and Rural Mental Health

Narcotics Anonymous (NA) offers a fellowship and support network for individuals recovering from substance use disorders. (https://www.na.org)

Rural Minds addresses mental health disparities in rural communities by providing resources. https://www.ruralminds.org

Comprehensive Coalitions and Initiatives

Mental Health America (MHA) leads the nation in community-based advocacy, public education, and connecting individuals with resources to improve mental wellness. (https://www.mhanational.org/)

The Mental Health Coalition is a collaborative initiative uniting mental health organizations to change awareness. (https: www.thementalhealthcoalition.org)

Bring Change to Mind raises awareness and encourages open dialogue about mental health to erase stigma. (https://www.bringchange2mind.org/)

Academic and Policy Resources

American Academy of Child and Adolescent Psychiatry (AACAP) provides resources to support the mental health of children and adolescents through education and clinical practice. (https://www.aacap.org/)

The National Association of School Psychologists (NASP) advocates for the development of school-based mental health services and policies. https://www.nasponline.org)

Family and Suicide Prevention

The National Federation of Families (NFF) empowers families with lived experience to influence mental health care policies and practices. (https://www.nasponline.org/)

Family Aware provides programs and resources to prevent depression and suicide among families. (https://www.familyaware.org/)

Holistic Well-Being and Mental Health Trusts

Well Being Trust is dedicated to advancing mental, social, and spiritual health for all by promoting a well-being framework. (https://www.wellbeingtrust.org/)

Each organization contributes to the mental health landscape, ensuring diverse needs are met with tailored support.

Index

A
Accepting our children for who they are, 85–103
Acknowledging the problem, 5, 6
Active listening, 7, 37, 48, 52, 54, 66, 74–76, 79, 83, 84
ADHD and DMDD, 20–21
Amantadine (Medication), 28–30, 47, 68, 122, 125, 144, 214
Anger, sudden fits of, 2, 53
Anika's story, 2–6, 9, 37, 38, 41, 42, 45, 46, 60–63, 68, 71–73, 75, 77, 79, 81, 82, 84, 87–93, 95, 96, 98, 99, 102, 106, 108, 110, 112–114, 119–121, 126–128, 130, 133, 135–137, 140, 141, 146, 147, 153, 154, 158, 162, 167, 168, 170, 171, 178, 179, 182, 183, 185, 186
Anxiety disorders and DMDD, 22
Attachment and emotional regulation, 16–19, 24, 25, 27, 31, 32, 55, 58, 71, 75, 78, 81, 94, 102, 107, 109–112, 115, 116, 123, 128, 129, 132, 151, 157, 162, 165–168, 170–172, 174, 177, 189–191, 194, 200, 206, 207, 217, 218, 221, 228
Autism spectrum disorder (ASD) and DMDD, 24–25

B
Barry's story, 85–87
Behavioral expectations, setting realistic, 38–39, 85–103, 111, 113
Boundaries, setting compassionate, 84
Brainstorming solutions, 146, 157–158

C
Celebrating small victories, 34, 39, 48, 56, 103
Challenges to acceptance, 97–101
Chronic irritability, 12, 22–25, 33, 35, 74
Cognitive-behavioral therapy (CBT), 9, 25, 31, 189–190
Communication, effective, 7, 34, 37, 38, 48, 68–84
Community service and social responsibility, 7, 9, 45, 46, 183
Community support, 10, 213
Compassionately addressing difficulties, 94–95
Compassion, developing, 8, 45–46, 177–188
Contributing factors to DMDD, 17–20
Co-occurring problems in DMDD, 20–25
Creating emotional safe havens, 96
Creating predictable routines, 89–90

D
Decision-making, teaching, 43, 144, 151, 157
Defining emotional dysregulation, 6, 183
Developing responsibility and compassion, 46
Developmental roots of DMDD, 15–16
Discipline, effective, 8, 43, 165, 166, 168, 170, 175
Disciplining for self-worth, 8, 43–45, 159–160
Disruptive mood dysregulation disorder (DMDD), definition, 12, 23
DMDD diagnosis, 21, 22, 198

E

Early childhood development and DMDD, 16
Early interventions, 15, 20, 32–34
Educational support, 52, 236
Emotional dysregulation, 6, 14, 16, 17, 19–21, 25, 31, 32, 55, 79, 98, 102, 107, 117, 126–128, 135, 137, 145, 149, 161, 166, 173, 175, 183, 189, 195, 210, 213, 221
Emotional exhaustion and burnout, 97–98
Emotional toll on families, 4, 211
Empathy, modeling by parentsc, 53
Empathy, teaching, 53–56
Environmental factors and DMDD, 14, 17–19, 27, 32
Exercises for problem-solving and decision-making, 149–151
Expressing affection through nonverbal cues, 88–89

F

Family dynamics, 5, 10, 23, 32, 66, 74, 79, 83, 84, 212
Final thoughts and cautionary notes, 47–49
Flexible parenting strategies, 49
Fostering a supportive environment, 95–97

G

Genetic factors in DMDD, 17
Guideposts, eight principles, 7, 9, 10, 35–49
Guilt, parental, 13, 63, 210

H

Helping children learn from mistakes, 135–139
Holistic approach to treatment, 33
Hope, the power of, 220

I

Identifying and reinforcing strengths, 93
Implications for treatment, 25–33
Importance of problem-solving skills, 164
Individualized education plan (IEP), 32, 67, 190–192, 195, 197, 199, 204
Intermittent explosive disorder (IED) and DMDD, 24
Irritability, managing, 24
Islands of competence, nurturing, 8, 40, 105–124

J

Jonas's story, 35–36
Joseph's story, 143–145

K

Kellan's story, 125–127, 139–140

L

Learning when to act, 216–217
Liam's story, 145

M

Major depression and DMDD, 23
Matthews protocol (treatment), 26, 28–31, 47, 86, 100, 102, 122, 125, 144, 159, 177, 190, 213–216
Medication, role of, 27, 214–215
Meltdowns in public, managing, 99–102
Mistakes, learning from, 131–132, 139
Modeling emotional regulation, 78–79, 84
Mood disorders, 6, 12, 15, 17, 18, 20, 21, 23, 31, 64, 144, 221

N

Nathan's story, 159–160
Navigating DMDD, 39, 48, 198
Neurobiological factors in DMDD, 17
Nurturing "Islands of Competence", 8, 40–41, 105–124
Nurturing strengths, 120–122

O

Obstacles to problem-solving, 151–154
Open communication, encouraging, 97
Oppositional defiant disorder (ODD) and DMDD, 22–23
Outbursts, intense emotional, 9, 52, 60, 74, 194, 220, 221

P

Parenting strategies, ineffectiveness, 5, 210
Parent-school partnership, establishing, 189–207
Parents, dreams and wishes of, 220–221
Patrick's story, 51–53, 219
Perspective-taking, encouraging, 58

Index

Pharmacotherapy for DMDD, 25, 27, 33
Positive reinforcement, 2, 7, 8, 32, 39, 44, 58, 93, 109, 117, 118, 129, 153, 166–167, 169, 172–174, 191, 200
Practical exercises for problem-solving, 149–151
Problem-solving, 8, 31, 42, 43, 58, 68, 71, 75, 108, 112, 127, 128, 132–134, 136, 143–158, 161, 164, 165, 171, 172, 176, 186–187, 191, 205, 216, 221, 225
Professional help, 5, 63
Public meltdowns and social stigma, 99–102

R
Raising resilient children, 7–9, 53–56
Reflective listening, 95, 98, 170
Reflective parenting practices, 182
Resilient children with DMDD, 7–9, 35–49, 68, 217–220
Responsibility, teaching, 8, 45, 185–188
Returning to Barry, 101–102
Returning to Bella and Lizzie, 69–70
Rising through the storm, 209–223

S
School-based intervention, 32, 33
Seeking help, first steps, 5–6
Self-care for parent, 52
Setting limits with compassion, 77
Setting realistic expectations, 7, 38–39, 48, 71, 85–103, 111–113
Siblings, impact on, 13
Social conscience, developing, 8, 45–46, 177–188
Storytelling and empathy, 52, 59, 60, 66, 93
Strategies for parents, 2–3, 64, 213
Supportive relationships, 7, 66, 215–216

T
Teachers, role in DMDD support, 129
Teaching empathy and compassion, 71
Temper tantrums *vs.* DMDD, 13, 24
Therapy, family and individual, 32
Treatment approaches, 20, 25, 177

W
Weighing pros and cons, 158
When ordinary parenting strategies fail, 2–3
Working with schools, 195

GPSR Compliance

The European Union's (EU) General Product Safety Regulation (GPSR) is a set of rules that requires consumer products to be safe and our obligations to ensure this.

If you have any concerns about our products, you can contact us on

ProductSafety@springernature.com

In case Publisher is established outside the EU, the EU authorized representative is:

Springer Nature Customer Service Center GmbH
Europaplatz 3
69115 Heidelberg, Germany

www.ingramcontent.com/pod-product-compliance
Lightning Source LLC
LaVergne TN
LVHW010338260326
834688LV00036B/762